ASPECTS OF FORENSIC PSYCHIATRIC NURSING

Aspects of Forensic Psychiatric Nursing

Edited by

PAUL MORRISON
PHILIP BURNARD
University of Wales College of Medicine

Avebury

Aldershot · Brookfield USA · Hong Kong · Singapore · Sydney

© P. Morrison and P. Burnard 1992

1000623134

Published by
Avebury
Ashgate Publishing Limited
Gower House
Croft Road
Aldershot
Hants GU11 3HR
England

Ashgate Publishing Company
Old Post Road
Brookfield
Vermont 05036
USA

A CIP catalogue record for this book is available from the British Library and the US Library of Congress

ISBN 1 85628 371 2

Printed and Bound in Great Britain by
Athenaeum Press Ltd., Newcastle upon Tyne.

Contents

Introduction

Paul Morrison and Philip Burnard

Forensic psychiatric nursing is a specialist branch of psychiatric nursing. Because the field is so new and because it is expanding rapidly, little research has been done in the field. Here we report a collection of small scale studies aimed at identifying some of the issues that need to be clarified in the field. Also included in this volume are some discussion and theory papers. We do not claim that they are exhaustive in their coverage - indeed they are highly selective. But when few research findings are available at all then it is important that such studies are published.

This book represents a beginning. All these chapters can do is to identify some of the factors that could be explored further. One thing is certain: a great deal of research needs to be done to lift the cloud of confusion that currently hovers over the field of forensic psychiatric nursing. Not least is the need to clarify the role of the forensic psychiatric nurse and, in particular, the specialist skills which are needed to fulfil the role effectively. As we shall see, there is often a tension between their current therapeutic orientation and their role as social policeman. We reiterate that these are preliminary studies. What is notable in all of them is a commitment on the part of forensic psychiatric nurses to find their own voice and their own role.

1 An historical and personal view of forensic nursing services

Barry Topping-Morris

The care and control of criminal, dangerous or difficult mentally ill patients has always been a problem for society. This problem then becomes a dilemma for nurses, for they need to combine caring with the need to ensure the continuing protection of the public. This nursing activity is referred to, in modern times, as Forensic Psychiatric Nursing and it takes place across a broad range of care provisions. These range from care in the community, through a gradation of secure provision to care under conditions of maximum security. This chapter explores the developments that have had an impact on Forensic Psychiatric Nursing throughout the United Kingdom during the last three decades.

The client group, in forensic nursing, is doubly stigmatised in as much as clients are both suffering from a mental illness and have offended in a manner that often proves distasteful to the general public at large. Such stigmatisation does not stop there, for mentally disordered offenders, detained under the Mental Health Act and in need of treatment or rehabilitation in a secure environment will often encounter a process of depersonalisation. The patient will often find that a label is attached, the definition and interpretation of which will prove to be crucial to future progress. They will have little opportunity to help to formulate these conclusions and the power to define who they are, will largely pass to others. Institutional life will determine who the patient will live with, what privacy they will have, if any; whether they will be at risk of assault from others around them; who will be allowed to visit them and how frequently; and how, if at all, they are able to express their own individuality and sexuality. They will fast become aware that information is being gathered about them, by others and without the surety that the content will be accurate in detail. The patient may discover that some types of behaviour, non-co-operation with treatment schedules, aggressive displays of anger or frustration, may be even leading to an assault, or an intense or suicidal mood will cause staff to separate them from other clients and they may come to interpret this as punishment for letting their feelings get out of control. This patient is likely to realise that there will be very little opportunity to vent these feelings without attracting some sort of sanction. Should the patient be fortunate enough to progress sufficiently so as to demonstrate to doctors and other staff that they could and should leave the institution, they may find that carers remain powerless to arrange such discharge until others co-operate.

Treatment provided in forensic settings is classically delivered by a very powerful 'institution' to a very powerless 'patient' - and the word here has more force than that of 'client' which is strongly suggestive of an equal relationship based on negotiated agreement, not on a status giving others the right to control (Bynoe, 1991). 'To deprive the individual in this case of his liberty for his own protection or to compel treatment involves a grave infringement of personal rights which must be subject to strict controls (Bluglass, 1983).

The concept of Regional Secure Unit provision originated in 1957 when the report of the Royal Commission proposed that dangerous patients should be accommodated in a few hospitals having suitable facilities for their treatment and custody. Some months prior to the 1959 MHA, the Ministry issued a warning against indiscriminate application of the open door principle, advising that there were some patients - not all of them having been before the courts - for whom the maintenance of adequate security precautions must be regarded as an essential part of their hospital care, either in their own interest or that of the community.

The first major milestone within the history was the implementation of the 1959 MHA which brought with it revolutionary changes; it allowed for the majority of the mentally disturbed to be admitted informally and it abolished most of the statutory distinctions between mental illness and mental deficiency. With regard to secure provision, the environment within which the principles of Forensic Psychiatric Nursing are most often practised, Section 97 obliged the Minister of Health to provide institutions for persons who 'require treatment under conditions of special security on account of their dangerous, violent or criminal propensities'. The 1959 Act was one of the first pieces of legislation that signalled the need to embrace the principal of community care within the spectrum of care provisions for the mentally ill. The Act was widely hailed as a most liberal reform which coincided with the developing 'open door' policy for psychiatric hospitals. According to Bluglass, it improved the acceptability of psychiatric care and reduced without entirely eliminating the stigma attached to it (Bluglass, in Gostin, 1985).

It soon became clear, however, that there was a group of patients in need of a type of care not falling within the philosophy of the open door regimes of many psychiatric hospitals. Consequently, in 1959, the then Minister of Health, Enoch Powell, appointed a working party to consider the provision of security in psychiatric hospitals and special hospitals. It reported in July 1961 and the report welcomed the open door principle but was convinced that security arrangements should continue in some regional NHS psychiatric hospitals. The problem for patients who had become known as the difficult and/or dangerous was that the majority of psychiatric hospitals claimed to have implemented a totally open door policy and felt that the hospital regime would be undermined by providing special care arrangements for a relatively limited group of patients at the expense of the remainder. Given that a change was taking place within psychiatry from the custodial to the therapeutic community concept, the 1961 proposal to provide security arrangements within Regional Health Authorities proved to be unattractive given that psychiatry was enthusiastic to rid itself of its victorian heritage.

The pioneering forensic psychiatrists which included Dr Peter Scott, Sir Dennis Hill and Professor Robert Bluglass, clearly recognised the consequences of this new movement and recognised that it was inappropriate for us to dismiss the importance of exercising security precautions, for those psychiatric patients that needed it given that security formed a very necessary part of treatment for the sake of the patients as well as the general public. They regarded the maximum secure provision found within the special hospital system as being cumbersome in that it did not best meet the needs of patients who should be offered more suitable arrangements which would enable treatment to occur closer to their own homes.

By the 1960's in the United Kingdom however, it was apparent that the open door policy of mental hospitals and the wholly commendable trend towards voluntary rather than compulsory admission to hospital for psychiatric treatment, was resulting in a neglect of a certain section of the mentally disordered population. The special hospitals such as Broadmoor, providing for treatment of patients in conditions of maximum security were now very overcrowded. Patients were being detained in those hospitals for longer than was necessary. On the other hand, open door modern psychiatric hospitals had no longer the facilities to cope with those patients who needed a degree of security in their management albeit a lesser degree than maximum. All too often, these patients ended up in prison, which became the only form of asylum available to them, there to be cared for more or less humanely by prison officers who had no training whatsoever in the treatment, management and nursing of mentally disordered people. Now the way in which we deal with all mentally disordered citizens and particularly how we deal with the mentally disordered offender, is a barometer of our civilisation. In spite of much vivid and enlightened legislation, it remains true that our chronically mentally disordered offenders are still given short shrift throughout much of the western world. Neither the mentally disordered nor the criminal is likely to be top of anyone's popularity list when it comes to portioning out limited resources, so not surprisingly this group has fared ill for many years. (Hunter, 1989).

There can be few sights more dispiriting than that of an acutely mentally ill man or woman incarcerated in a modern prison, in Britain, today. Such a person must suffer very deeply, must experience very real mental pain, which is as much deserving of our attention, sympathy and treatment as the man with a physical disorder..

Faced with increasing numbers of such people ending up in prison, there were 2 reports commissioned in the early 1970's, one into secure provision in the NHS called The Glancy Report and the other more widely targeting all aspects of the problems posed to society by the mentally abnormal offender called The Butler Report.

5

In 1973 the then Department of Health and Social Security in its memorandum, Hospital Services for the Mentally Ill (DHSS, 1971 a) reiterated departmental policy that the NHS should provide some security arrangements. In the same year a departmental working party was set up under the Chairmanship of Dr Glancy to review the existing guidance on security in NHS psychiatric hospitals and to make recommendations on the present and future need for such security. Reporting in March, 1974 the Glancy working party found that most hospitals were expected to make their own arrangements for dealing with difficult patients, which usually consisted of one or two locked wards integrated with generic psychiatry. This report recommended immediate planning for 1,000 secure beds at regional level, a formula approximating to 20 beds per million of the catchment population.

Four months later in July 1974 the Committee on Mentally Abnormal Offenders (Butler Committee, 1974) published an interim report stressing the urgency of providing regional secure units. They described a yawning gap between NHS hospitals with no secure provision and the overcrowded special hospitals. Such absence of intermediate security, together with the development of treatment in open conditions in local hospitals was having adverse affects on the special hospitals, the criminal justice system and the prisons. The Butler Committee found that the special hospitals felt obliged to accept dangerous psychiatric patients from the open psychiatric hospitals but were experiencing difficulties in transferring patients back to the open psychiatric hospitals who were deemed no longer dangerous. The courts were finding it increasingly difficult to secure a psychiatric bed for mentally disordered offenders and even when such a bed was available the lack of security often mitigated against such a placement. For such offenders, unless they satisfied a criteria for admission to a special hospital the courts often had no alternative other than to seek a penal disposal. Meanwhile, evidence was given to The Butler Committee of the growing number of mentally disordered people found within the prison establishments. Not only were mentally abnormal offenders imprisoned for want of a hospital bed, but the prisons were unable to transfer its own inmates to NHS resources whenever they became mentally disordered whilst serving their sentences.

The Butler Committee recommended a target figure of 2,000 secure places to meet the needs of the NHS, the special hospitals, the courts and the prison, a formula approximating to 40 beds per million of the catchment population. In July 1974 the then Secretary of State Barbara Castle announced the governments acceptance of the recommendations of the interim report of The Butler Committee and The Glancy Report and declared that 1,000 secure places were to be provided in the first instance. In accepting the interim report of The Butler Committee the Government made capital money available from central funds to build permanent units and to fund interim secure units as a temporary solution. The DHSS provided design guidelines which indicated the Governments view on their design and discussed the proposed patients, treatment, commented on the disturbing lack of progress in setting up regional secure units. In 1976 the DHSS made a special revenue allocation to each regional health authority to cover a proportion of the staffing costs. In 1982, the details of the cash allocations made to regional health authorities was published (Hansard, 1982) and the disturbing fact emerged that not all revenue expenditure had found its way into psychiatric services let alone into secure facilities.

It was not until November 1980 that the first regional secure unit began admitting patients and it then took over $2\frac{1}{2}$ years for a further 3 units to open. The estimate of 20 beds in The Glancy Report presumably being chosen in preference to the 40 beds per million of The Butler Report because it was smaller and cheaper and not because any convincing research had been done to estimate the size of the problem. Despite this criticism, what the Butler and Glancy Reports really did was to pump money and political influence into forensic psychiatry services. How this was to be handled in each region was left to each regional health authority and what has actually happened has varied very much, not least of all determined by whether the region had a product champion in post, whether he/she was continually present, was really interested in patient work, what sort of planner, politician and manager he/she was, or what the opposition was like and whether the fates smiled upon them. It is worthy of note, that medical staff are often elevated to the status of 'production champion' but this sadly, fails to recognise the depth of contribution made by nursing's 'product champions' eg, Parry, Hillis, Tait and Hendry to mention but a few.

Many will be familiar with the pace (or in some instances lack of pace) of debate and developments that immediately followed the Glancy and Butler Reports of the 1970's At this stage it would be easy for me to enter into the debate and comment on the effect these reports had on developments, but instead I would prefer to reflect on our apparent inability to respond to the warning signs given in 1957 and more importantly the seemingly irreparable damage done to psychiatry's attitude towards the difficult patient.

The approximate 20 year gap between the warning signs in 1957 and the opening of the country's first interim secure unit at Rainhill Hospital Merseyside in August 1976, brought about a seriously damaging change of attitude, with far reaching consequences that are being encountered as we move towards the mid 90's. The inclinations, interest, skills and abilities to manage the difficult patient, left our profession as quickly as did its patients through the open door towards the community. This was the conception of the 'yawning gap' referred to in The Butler Report which in subsequent years was to mature and compromise our special hospitals, the criminal justice system and the prison populations. The special hospitals felt obliged to accept dangerous psychiatric patients from the open hospitals but experienced difficulty in transferring back into the open hospitals patients who were no longer difficult or dangerous. The courts found difficulty obtaining NHS beds for mentally abnormal offenders due jointly to a reluctance amongst clinicians and an absence of secure accommodation. Such offenders failing to meet criteria for admission to special hospitals were often given a prison disposal.

From the beginning of the 19th Century it has been recognised that the quality of nursing care is directly associated with security and that physical security as such tends to militate against the exercise of proper nursing practise. In 1813 Samuel Tuke, grandson of William Tuke who founded the retreat at York, wrote:

> In the construction of asylums, cure and comfort ought to be as much considered as security, and I have no hesitation in declaring that a system which, by limiting the power of the attendant, obliges him not to neglect his duty, makes it his interest to obtain the good opinion of those under his care, provides more effectually for the safety of the keeper, as well as of the patient, than all the apparatus of chains, darkness and anodynes (Tuke, 1813).

The physical confinement of patients, however brought about, is for the protection of the public, but secure institutions also have their responsibility to protect both staff and patients within the establishments and such internal aspects of security coincide with and are indistinguishable from the wider organisational requirements for control. Aspects of internal security may include, as in the special hospital, the frequent counting and searching of patients, the monitoring of the movement of patients around the hospital by centralized radio contact and the use of drugs as a means of controlling violent and disruptive patients. Seclusion and latterly, Control and Restraint have subsequently assumed a disproportionate relevance in the management of behavioural extremes, and will be discussed in greater detail later in this chapter.

Government policy on mentally disordered offenders pursues the basic principal that, where possible, they should receive care and treatment in hospital from health and social services rather than in the criminal justice system.

The Governments objective is to ensure that we have a just and humane system, providing the most up to date methods of care and treatment for such people. In practice -

- This means ensuring that people defined by the Mental Health Act as liable to be detained, who are brought before the courts, are directed from the penal system to hospital. This should be before or at the initial hearing or, failing that, from Prison to Hospital as soon as the need arises.

- It means the Government and Health Authorities continuing to work to ensure that the NHS is able to accommodate such patients and that a comprehensive service and an adequate range of secure facilities is available.

- It also means seeking to achieve more sensitive and flexible referral mechanisms and encouraging effective collaboration between professional staff, health, and Social Service bodies, and the Criminal Justice System. Collaboration must encompass strategic service planning as well as day to day work.

Many will be aware of the changes in services for mentally disordered offenders since the Butler and Glancy reports in the mid 1970's, but it is worth reiterating a few initiatives to show just how far we have come over the last 15 years or so. They include:

> The establishment of the Regional Secure Unit programme, with central funding, and subsequent action by Health Authorities to provide a network of units offering treatment over a period of one to two years for those requiring treatment in security less intense than that offered by the Special Hospitals. Thirteen regions now have an RSU, and proposals are currently being considered from the fourteenth. In all over fifty million pounds at today's prices has been spent on Regional Secure Unit capital development. However, there is no doubt that the RSU programme has taken far longer to implement than was originally anticipated and that even now there would appear to be scope for further expansion of regionally based secure provision although not necessarily with an RSU focus (Dorrell, 1991).

These initiatives, combined with effective local planning in a number of areas, have helped produce a much improved range of services for mentally disordered offenders. At the most secure level there are three Special Hospitals, with places for about 1,700 detained patients. There is then the medium security of the RSU's with about 650 beds. Locally, there exists about 35,000 mental illness and 30,000 mental handicapped beds, including some 2,000 beds (albeit not all for offenders) on so called 'locked' or partially locked wards.

Complimentary to these services are, the community based services. These will receive a boost from the introduction of the 'care programme' initiative in 1992. The initiative is designed to provide systematic arrangements for the health and social care of vulnerable patients outside hospital, and should help to reduce the number of patients 'falling out' from care into dereliction and crime.

Over the last two decades, Forensic Psychiatry has come to be recognised as a specialty in its own right. It has developed rapidly with the appointment of consultants and advisors in every health region.In October 1989 the Special Hospital Service Authority was established.

The SHSA now exercises its responsibilities through general managers at hospital level, but remains accountable to the Secretary of State for Health. Giving local managers new responsibilities and greater freedom to run Special Hospitals has improved the management of the service and reduced its isolation from the rest of the NHS.

These are all very positive developments, but they are just a start. There remains great potential and great need for further progress in this difficult arena. Some mentally disordered offenders, for example, remain in unsuitable placements, people in Prison who should be in hospital, others in maximum secure provision who need a less secure regime. There is undoubtedly under provision of a suitable range of accommodation in certain areas, for example, of longer term medium secure facilities.

Some professionals claim that many of the problems now facing the criminal justice system and the prisons have been caused by the long standing Governmental policy, to which they remain committed, of moving from a service based mainly on large mental hospitals to more local services comprising of both in-patient services and care in the community. The perceived inadequacies of care in the community are blamed for allowing neglected people to drift into crime; a perceived shortage of beds is blamed for their incarceration in prison.

It is certainly true that the number of patients in long stay hospitals has been falling in this country since the mid 1950's -as they have been in virtually all other developed countries. In 1976 there were some 84,000 patients in mental illness hospitals and 49,000 in mental handicapped hospitals; by 1986 there were 60,000 and 34,000 respectively.

Within the remaining psychiatric services there are at present some 2,000 beds in wards that are or can be locked. At the time of the Butler and Glancy reports there were some 13,000 locked or lockable beds; yet the problems then were very similar to the problems now.

While the numbers of people in hospital have fallen, the growth of facilities outside hospital has continued a pace; there has been a virtual doubling of residential facilities for mentally ill adults; an increase in social services day care for the same group; and an increase in NHS day patient care. Activity levels and overall expenditure on mental illness provision has increased, as have the numbers of key professional staff. Hospital and community health service expenditure on mental

11

illness is still concentrating very largely on in-patient provision. So, the above suggests that far more lies behind the problems of ensuring proper services for mentally disordered offenders than simply a decrease in hospital beds.

That is not to say, that the balance or range of provision for the mentally ill is necessarily right. The development of community care in particular has not kept pace everywhere with the demands made upon it. The Government are introducing the 'care programme' approach, to offset this imbalance. A central feature of such a care programme is that mentally ill people in need of specialised care should be offered such, as in-patients if services are not yet available in the community.

Review of services for mentally disordered offenders in England

On the 30th November 1990 a review of the current level, pattern, and operation of health and social services for mentally disordered offenders in England was announced by Stephen Dorrell, Parliamentary Secretary for Health.

The joint Department of Health and Home Office Steering Committee will decide where changes are needed for the existing system, and how any changes might be brought about. The Committee is expected to complete its work by the autumn of 1992. The review is expected to pursue the basic principal of government policy today, that is, where possible, mentally disordered offenders should receive care and treatment in hospital from Health and Social Services, rather than in the Criminal Justice System.

This will require that we should ensure that people defined by the Mental Health Act as liable to be detained, who are brought before the courts, are directed from the penal system to hospital. Further, it will require the government and Health Authorities to continue to work together to ensure that the NHS is able to accommodate such patients, and that a comprehensive service and an adequate range of secure facilities is available.

The Steering Committee has a membership which includes officials from the Department of Health and the Home Office, from the Health and Social Services, the Special Hospitals Service Authority, and the Criminal Justice System. The review is expected to look at present arrangements for funding service developments and their possible improvement. The review is also expected to consider relevant research and other studies. The review is primarily concerned with services in England, but Wales, Scotland and Northern Ireland will maintain an interest in its progress.The review will be concerned essentially with assessing how services should be developed within the framework of existing legislation. It is not intended as a review of the law, given that parliament went to great lengths in 1983 to strike the right balance between the interests of patients and their families, and the community at large.

The professions believe that the review will offer a real prospect of addressing in depth many of the important issues that confront those concerned with the health and welfare of mentally disordered offenders. They consider the work to be of great importance.

Although the number of mentally disordered offenders is still relatively small, they nonetheless achieve a high profile by virtue of the multiplicity of health and social problems that they present.

As well as having a mental disorder and having offended, some of those patients coming from prison, the courts and the Special Hospitals have also misused drugs or alcohol, or may have been homeless or unemployed.

The patients have often come to expect little from the community. It has, therefore, been - and remains - a significant task to adapt our services in this area to modern methods of care and treatment, and ideas of what is just and humane. The terms of reference of the Steering Committee are: To plan, co-ordinate and direct a review of the Health and Social Services provided in England by the NHS, SHSA, and Local Authorities for mentally disordered offenders (and others requiring similar services without having come before the courts), with a view to determining whether changes are needed in the current level, pattern, or operation of services and identifying ways of promoting such changes, having regard to:

- The development of new management arrangements in the NHS and the proposals for development of community care.

- The implications for NHS Forensic Psychiatry of action to follow up the report of the Home Office efficiency scrutiny on the prison medical service.

- Any relevant recommendations of the inquiry into the Strangeways Prison disturbances (the Woolf inquiry and other prison related inquiries).

- Present arrangements for funding services and service developments, and their possible improvement.

- Relevant research and studies.

- This review offers an excellent opportunity to address in detail many of the important issues that confront those concerned for the health and welfare of mentally disordered offenders. It will be important work, forming part of the government's strategy to improve the range and effectiveness of services for people needing specialised treatment and care. The issues are challenging. They call for sustained and imaginative commitment on the part of many people working in a multi-plicity of agencies (Dorrell, 1990).

Regionalised Forensic Psychiatric Services despite having a 16 year history, nonetheless, remain in their earliest developmental stages. As a consequence of this delicate stage, the services require special protection and the RCN have been urged to pressure the Reed Committee to consider the following:

- Adequate funding for the further development of the Forensic Psychiatric Service at a regional level should continue to be provided centrally by the Department of Health but with the introduction of a mechanism that will ensure that the funding reaches its intended source.

- Regionalised Forensic Psychiatric Services should be provided evenly across the United Kingdom and should be funded outside the new internal market being set within the NHS at least for the foreseeable future by describing special protection.

- There should be closer working relationships between the Special Hospitals and the Regional Secure Services designed to ensure an easier exchange of patients between the two services with added emphasis on obtaining more suitable, less secure placements outside of Special Hospital for those patients currently inappropriately detained under conditions of maximum security.

- If HC66/90 is to achieve its necessary effect in enabling mentally disordered offenders to be diverted away from the criminal justice system then the Reed Committee might be best advised to eliminate current confusion that abounds, as to who's responsibility it actually is to bring about the diversion, is it generic psychiatry's responsibility or the Forensic Specialty's remit? Either way adequate funding will be called for.

- The Reed Committee should seriously consider the therapeutic validity of our more aged Special Hospitals and in the very least actively encourage the same institutions to philosophically update themselves.

- Generally speaking, co-ordination and integration of services for mentally disordered offenders across the whole spectrum of provision, from the criminal justice system, through the Forensic Specialty provision and within the community are sadly lacking. The Reed committee might seek to somehow draw this together by introducing a means to ensure monitoring and evaluation of the whole provision takes place regularly.

- Little if any provision has been made for difficult to manage patients or mentally disordered offenders who need services offering less security than the RSU programme. Wherever hospitals have already been de-centralised and closed, how will the Reed Committee propose to ensure that the District Health Authorities revisit the need to provide difficult to place and intensive care units services where necessary.

- Is there a place for mentally disordered offenders in the criminal justice system long term? Perhaps mentally disordered offenders should only interface with the criminal justice system until such time as disposal is finalised.

- In every region there should be a Forensic Psychiatric Nurse Advisor to assist and promote developments, their contribution is just as worthy as the medical contribution. There should be a formal mechanism for linking Health Authority Developments for this disadvantaged client group with the role of the advisors.

- Basic training for Psychiatric Nurses needs to reflect a greater input from and emphasis on, Forensic Psychiatric Nursing.

How will the department of health regularly monitor capacity, will monitoring be linked with regional advisory roles (to include nursing)? The quality and type of place available needs to monitored as well as the capacity. But, more importantly, will the 'monitors' have the power to instigate change?

In 1813 Samuel Tuke first warned of the importance of the client centred approach, the Percy Commission in 1957 forecast difficulties on the horizon, the Glancy and Butler Reports of the early 70's identified the need for specialist service provision, and yet here we are in 1992 eagerly awaiting the Reed Committee's final recommendations on how best to respond to the needs of mentally disordered offenders. If the patient sits comfortably in the midst of these anticipated deliberations, then we might just get it right this time?

Code of practice

The guidance within the code is intended primarily to accommodate the needs, rights and entitlements of mentally disordered persons who are detained under relevant mental health legislation. However, much of the code is equally applicable to informal patients and practitioners should seek to ensure the code is equally available to, and referred to as, a good practice document for the care and management of all mentally disordered patients. This, of course, includes mentally disordered offenders, the code's principles and guidelines are of particular relevance to this client group given that almost always, the client is compulsorily detained. Chapters one, three, seven, ten, twelve, fifteen and eighteen are of particular relevance to the mentally disordered offender.

The Mental Health Act 1983 does not impose a legal duty to comply with the code but failure to follow the code could be referred to in evidence in legal proceedings. Unfortunately, in practice, the code is often used as a reference book, the user visiting the index to seek the subject area of particular relevance. This often results in the code's broad principles being overlooked and with this point in mind it is worthwhile to visit these principles. All people being assessed for possible admission under the Act or to whom the Act applies should:

- Receive respect for and consideration of their individual qualities and diverse background - social, cultural, ethnic and religious.

- Have their needs taken fully into account though it is recognised that, within available resources, it may not always be practicable to meet them.

- Be delivered any necessary treatment or care in the least controlled and segregated facilities practicable.

- Be treated or cared for in such a way that promotes to the greatest practicable degree, their self determination and personal responsibility consistent with their needs and wishes.

- Be discharged from any order under the Act to which they are subject immediately it is no longer necessary.

This means that patients should be as fully involved as practicable, consistent with their needs and wishes, in the formulation and delivery of care and treatment. It means that patients should have their legal rights drawn to their attention, consistent with their capacity to understand them.

Finally it means that, when treatment or care is provided in conditions of security, patients should be subject only to the level of security appropriate to their individual needs and only for so long as it is required (Code of Practice, 1990). What remains to be seen is whether or not, the practitioner can reflect this good will found within the code, in his/her everyday practice when caring for patients who present with particular management problems.

Forensic psychiatric nurses association

The FPNA was launched in 1987 at an inaugural meeting held at the Three Bridges Regional Secure Unit in Ealing, London. The need for the setting up of such a organisation had been debated by senior staff from a variety of regional services up and down the country, but the energies stemmed precisely from a 'meeting of minds', representative of views to be found within RSU's south of Watford Gap and RSU's north of Watford Gap. Forensic Psychiatric Services was growing in leaps and bounds in the mid 80's and much rivalry existed between RSU's, Special Hospitals and other services caring for the client group. This 'meeting of the minds' recognised the need for forensic psychiatric nurses to organise themselves within a professional body for many reasons;

- Firstly they considered themselves to be a specialist group of staff spread thinly throughout the country, with specific professional, educational and training needs which were unlikely to be met by any of other organisation.

- Secondly they were often affected by the decisions and the comments of other influential bodies, and to date had not had a representative voice which had gained general acceptance.

- Thirdly, they needed to share experience and expertise. Such a sharing could prove to be difficult without the framework of a national organisation to support it. The needs of the nursing staff working within such services were numerous and an association was desperately needed to clarify and then meet those needs.

An executive committee was appointed which included Mr Tony Hillis from the Reaside Clinic as its President with representatives drawn from other RSU's and including Stan King, Shaun Payne, John Kilshaw and Barry Topping-Morris. The association has since flourished with the help of some sterling efforts from the current Secretary Mr David Sallah. Such that it has staged four conferences to date all of which have been extremely stimulating whilst organising itself sufficiently to attract a membership from Special Hospitals, Regional Secure Units and Generic Psychiatry with associate membership being extended towards the other professions. It publishes a regular journal and I understand that this journal will soon be assuming a glossy format being published by an eminent publisher.

The association has emerged as a strong representative voice for the specialist nursing activity within the forensic domain and uses its influence as a recognised organisation to advise, support, and criticise national policy affecting mentally disordered offenders.

Later this year the FPNA is to hold a further conference at the NEC in Birmingham to which it has attracted a formidable list of speakers to include representation from the Mental Health Act Commission, the Reed Committee and distinguished speakers from the professions concerned with the client group. Its committee is to be much applauded for having grasped the nettle and taken on the responsibility of promoting services for this disadvantaged client group and it deserves to achieve much success, as am sure it will, over coming years.

Representative bodies of this specialty

An entity group exists within the Royal College of Nursing in the form of the Forum for Nurses Working within a Controlled Environment. Such national membership groups are a recognised and essential component of the work of the Royal College of Nursing, in that they facilitate communication and debate about nursing policy and practice. The aim of this Forum is to promote the recognition of the need for the ongoing development of controlled environments as an integral part of a comprehensive health service and to identify the contribution of nurses in all such component parts of that service. The Forum would wish to actively discourage the treatment and rehabilitation of mentally disordered persons in prisons or in environments other than those that offer recognised care. Prior to 1989 the Forum, then entitled the Forum for Nurses Working in a Secure Environment, was a subgroup of the Mental Health Nursing Society within the college and had been active since the late 1970's. The Forum now has its own executive committee, budget and control over its own affairs. The Forum hopes to achieve its aims by encouraging an exchange of national and international views and information of nursing in this specialty by contributing to the formulation of improved links between controlled and conventional psychiatric facilities. Furthermore, it would wish to promote and encourage research into the effects of providing assessment, treatment, rehabilitation and aftercare to the defined client group within the controlled environment.

As with all branches of nursing the relationship between nurse and patient is crucial. In a controlled environment not only is the nurse a friend, advocate and mentor, but often is the intermediary between the patient and society. A broad range of skills is required covering physical as well as psychological care and the client group will often be those who have displayed extremes of social deviance.

Some people because of their severe state of mental distress or because of offences committed or alleged, need to be given care in situations which call for greater supervision or security to compliment conventional psychiatric care. The balance between security and the provision of a therapeutic environment can present nurses with a serious dilemma. The need to ensure the continuing protection of the public often conflicts with the nurses role in ensuring that treatment and rehabilitation in secure conditions lasts for the minimum necessary period. The particular skills that allow nurses to cope with this often contradictory balance are represented in the Forum which is open to all RCN members who work in situations where security for the individual or for society at large, plays a complimentary role in care. Whether practising in locked environments, hospital settings or defined secure units for mentally ill or mentally impaired people. Whether in one of the special hospitals or a practising nurse within the prison nursing service, the Forum has something to offer you and conversely you have something to contribute to the challenges of the future that the Forum must face.

The Forum endeavours to promote the art and science of nursing within controlled environments by actively engaging itself in a wide range of specific issues of relevance to mentally disordered patients who find themselves in need of secure care.

The Forum is currently engaged in consultation with the wider profession regarding the use of seclusion, control and restraint within the mental health nursing domain. The use of seclusion, control and restraint is a major policy area affecting psychiatric nursing practice. The RCN's Forum for Nursing in a Controlled Environment has produced guidelines recently for consultation with the wider profession, with good practice indicators to assist both mental health care workers and other staff in statutory and health care settings to improve standards of practice within this sensitive arena. Following the consultation exercise the Forum will need to reproduce such guidelines and distribute them accordingly to interested parties.

The Forum is eager to critique the recommendations that will be forthcoming in the autumn of 1992 relating to the 'Review of Health and Social Services for Mentally Disordered Offenders'. Given that this is the most important review of services for mentally disordered offenders to occur in the United Kingdom post 1975, the Royal College of Nursing and the Forum will be eager to discuss and debate its content.

The Royal College of Nursing needs no reminding of the sensitivity of the work being conducted by the 'committee of enquiry into complaints about Ashworth Special Hospital'. Later this year it can be expected that the Chairman of the Committee of Inquiry Sir Louis Blom-Cooper will release its findings and recommendations to a wider audience. Given the sensitivity of this enquiry, together with the need to ensure college members currently nursing within special hospitals, are given every opportunity to flourish within this difficult domain, the Forum would wish to spend considerable time to consider the committees recommendations and the impact of the proposals on the client group/staff working within the special hospital.

The forthcoming year is a very crucial one for mental health nurses. In April 1992, Virginia Bottomley, Minister of Health, announced the Department of Health's Mental Health Nursing Review. The professions call for this mental health nursing review to be swift and desires that the membership of the review team must include investigators who will not fudge the facts or cover mistakes and past misjudgments. The Forum for Nurses Working in Controlled Environments intends to keep a very close eye indeed on these developments.

Control and restraint

In July 1984 a patient was found dead within a seclusion room in, Norfolk House, Broadmoor Special Hospital. Subsequently an inquiry was made into the circumstances surrounding the incident, to consider the care and treatment accorded to the patient before and during his seclusion on the said date and to report conclusions relating to the matter; and in the light of those conclusions to recommend any action that should be taken in relation to patient care. As a result of this inquiry a confidential report made the following recommendations:

- More qualified nursing staff and occupational therapists should be employed in order to improve the quality of life of patients and to prevent the build up of frustration in both patients and staff.

- Proper training in physical control and restraint of patients should be given to all nursing staff. The course recently introduced at Broadmoor should become a compulsory and regular part of nurse training at the hospital.

- The recently introduced guideline governing movement of patients within Norfolk House should continue to apply and staff should be reminded of it regularly.

- The decision to administer heavy sedatives should be made by a Doctor and not by nursing staff. The decision should be made at the time of the incident by a Doctor in attendance on the ward. He should be made fully aware of the extent of violence immediately preceding his attendance and of the quality and quantity of food recently consumed by the patient.

- Observation of the heavily sedated patient should be constant and should take place within the side room in which he is confined (Ritchie, 1984).

Since the above report in 1984 courses in Control and Restraint have been conducted at various locations throughout the United Kingdom by Home Office 'approved' instructors and are based on locally determined formats. No single body is responsible for the examination of the philosophy and content of these courses and no recognition is given to attendance on such courses by the statutory bodies. Control and restraint training was considered by the National Boards in 1988 whilst generating the outline curriculum for the ENB 770 course (Nursing within Controlled Environments). The National Boards then agreed that control and restraint training need not be included in the outline curriculum but that reference would be confined to an examination of such provision and the ethical issues generated. This decision was based on the fact that courses in control and restraint were available nationally and were the responsibility of local management as regards provision for the safety of staff placed in vulnerable circumstance.

During 1990 the National Board's received representation from a number of sources expressing concern that nurses, midwives and health visitors were vulnerable whilst undertaking their normal and required duties, due to the increase in violence within society. Subsequently, recommendation was made to the National Boards that, in view of the implication for nurses, midwives and health visitors and the views from the branches of the professions that a training need existed, the Board would establish a working group to examine the issues and make appropriate recommendations. The terms of reference of this working group was; 'to examine issues relevant to the provision of control and restraint training for nurses, midwives and health visitors and to make recommendations'.

The working group subsequently asked the National Board to consider and agree the following recommendations:

- That the Board issue a statement concerning the inclusion in all its approved preregistration courses of the opportunity to examine issues

23

relevant to the subject of violence in society and the management of anti-social behaviour.

- That the Board agreed to receive applications for the approval of courses in 'the management of anti-social behaviours'.

- That such courses be generated by educational institutions and be based on an intention guideline issues by the Board.

- That such courses be set at a minimum of 'certificate of competence' level and that local negotiation with higher education will determine the level of academic award.

- That such courses be concerned with the needs of the care delivery group.

- That the working group be reconvened for a further meeting to set and agree a statement outlining the intention of these courses.

- That the Board establish a small working group to examine in detail the training and approval of instructors in control and restraint techniques and make recommendations.

The English National Board has since considered and accepted the report of the Working Group and accepted all of the recommendations made with minor reservations. The Board considered that in the view of the need to examine certain issues in detail and to ensure that there is national comparability between courses, further work needs to be generated and undertaken by the Board. Such work would be placed within the terms of reference of a specialist panel who would be tasked with the responsibility of providing an outline curriculum and national guidance on the subject matter. Such a specialist panel has yet to be convened but there remains a strong expectation that an outline curriculum will be available in the latter months of 1992 (ENB, 1992).

Nurses are of the opinion that the 'professionalization' of control and restraint is long overdue, the profession desperately needs the guidelines that could be offered by the above specialist panel, The Guardian newspaper recently carried a story alleging that nine nursing staff from Rampton top security Hospital in Nottinghamshire had been arrested in connection with the death of a patient in late May of 1992. The newspaper reports that a second postmortem held on the deceased had lead to 'some concern about the restraint holds placed on the patient prior to his death'. This development comes at a time of controversy over the care of patients in the three English Special Hospitals at Rampton, Broadmoor in Berkshire and Ashworth on Merseyside. How much longer do nurses need to wait before they are offered the protection of a 'professionalised' course in control and restraint, made available to help allay nurses anxieties and to help prevent the above unfortunate circumstance recurring?

Educational initiatives

ENB 960

This course has been running in each of the special hospitals since the late 70's and was originally designed to enable experienced psychiatric nurses to make a positive contribution to therapeutic treatment programmes within a secure environment. The curriculum was originally designed to meet the needs of those nurses who were expected to care for mentally disordered offenders within conditions of medium security. The course would enable an appreciation of the philosophy of care to be developed within such environments, and to enable nurses to plan and develop the nursing component of a multidisciplinary approach to the management of therapeutic programmes within such units. The objectives of the course were as follows:

- To describe the rationale for providing a psychiatric service for patients exhibiting a degree of behavioural disturbance which required treatment within a secure unit.

- To incorporate appropriately, previously acquired psychiatric nursing skills in the therapeutic programmes developed for such a service.

- To make objective assessments of patients using the reported observations, written reports and any other assessment methods in current use.

- To participate in the formulation of treatment policies as part of a multidisciplinary team.

- To make an appraisal of implications of maintaining a level of security consistent with the treatment aims of the unit, observing the principals of being non-provocative in the application of control.

- To give an account of the relationship of this service to other services available for the management of the anticipated patient population eg those provided by the National Health Service, Local Authorities and the Home Office.

- To discuss the legal aspects of the rights and responsibilities of patients and staff within units providing a secure environment;

- To recognise individual and group attitudes to nursing and to formulate, adapt, and change attitudes that will enhance an understanding of patient needs and the quality of care in this specialty.

- To demonstrate the skills which develop, maintain and improve communication and to develop more self awareness and interpersonal skills in communicating with patients, relatives, colleagues and others.

- To appreciate the value and implications of nursing research findings and their application to nursing practices.

- To develop a systematic to assessing, planning, implementing and evaluating approach the organisation and management of nursing care in the secure environment.

- To appraise the organisational management of the clinical environment provided for patients nursed in a secure unit, taking into consideration the ethical aspects of the work with patients, relatives and staff.

- To develop further appreciation and understanding of the learning process and fundamental aspects of teaching patients, relatives, colleagues and others and to help recognise the necessity for ones own continuing educational and professional development (ENB, 1986).

It is ironic that although the course was to meet the educational needs of nurses expected to work within conditions of medium security the first course venues approved by the English National Board were in fact within the special hospitals. As early as 1980 ENB 960 course members were producing work which seriously questioned the wisdom of staging these courses within the special hospitals given that the special hospitals offered conditions of maximum security, whilst this new generation of nurses would be expected to nurse in conditions of medium security within regional secure units. The philosophy and practice differed immensely, thankfully, this new breed of nurse being generated, resisted all attempts to conform to the 'custodial' role, promoted the value of nursing using therapeutic security and good psychiatric nursing skills, to such a degree that I now believe it to be possible to provide the training within the MSU base, using these new venues as 'change agents' to improve practice within the special hospitals. Some may suggest this to be a radical proposal but I firmly believe that such a shift would bring about better protection and promotion of patient primacy principles.

Throughout the 1970's following the recommendations made by both the Glancy and the Butler reports a number of medium secure environments emerged providing specialist services for those patients who required very high standards of psychiatric nursing care under conditions of medium security. The pioneers in this infant specialty had to accommodate and adapt to a situation not previously faced by psychiatric nurses and were certainly not envisaged or provided for in the basic nurse training syllabus.

The situations in question included reassuring a fearful public and shaping and defining the nurses role in a truly multi-disciplinary setting, all the time attempting to emphasise the therapeutic role in a setting which clearly deprives the patients of their liberty. They had to seek a new identity within their own hospital and with colleagues with whom they had worked closely for many years. Consequently hopes and aspirations were often dashed, much to the dismay of the team leaders, but perhaps more significantly to the newly formed caring team who had built up hopes on behalf of their patients. However these adversities appear to have lead to the emergence of one common characteristic, that is, the eagerness of the experienced staff to share their knowledge and experience. No one would claim to have all the answers and clearly each unit developed its own distinct policies and practices which were kept under constant review. I believe that the Project 2000 branch programme for Mental Health would be best advised to include the above in its content, whilst the Review of Mental Health will surely need to recognise this important role played by Forensic psychiatric nurses.

ENB 955

The above course was first founded sometime in the late 1970's, it made its entry into the realms of post basic education for forensic psychiatric nursing at or about the same time as the ENB 960 course. The course was intended for those nurses whose names appeared on part one, two, three, four, five, six, seven, eight or ten of the UKCC active register. The rationale for the course was that violence was a way in which some people expressed their anger, fear or despair and that inevitably, most nurses would encounter this violence in the form of verbal aggression, threatening behaviour or physical assault on people or property. The course intended to provide nurses and midwives with the information required to deepen their knowledge and understanding of the aetiology of violence, preventative means of reducing its occurrence and a means of managing violence as and when it occurs, followed by the restoration of the status quo and a return to normality once the violent episode had ended. The aim of the course was to enable nurses and midwives to gain an increased awareness and understanding of internal and external factors which provoke aggressive and violent responses from patients and relatives, and develop appropriate skills in managing potential and actual violent behaviour.

28

This course proved to be very popular, it was attractive to the practitioner, sufficiently cheap enough for managers to invest in it, but perhaps most importantly, the course could be taken by students of other disciplines and this provided a very rich opportunity, taken by many, to address the issues facing society as a result of violence, in a multi-professional manner. Consequently, I would hope that any future courses generated should automatically include multi professional contribution and attendance.

ENB 770 COURSE

In November 1988 the National Boards for England and Wales produced an outline curriculum for 'Nursing within Controlled Environments'. The term 'controlled environments' was used to describe the wide spectrum of resources in which care and treatment is offered to people with mental illness and/or handicap who have offended, are likely to offend, or for management reasons, have been or remained subject to detention. Such environments include Special Hospitals, Regional Secure Units, Controlled NHS Hospital or Community Units, Home Office Administered Establishments and domiciliary and rehabilitation services related to these.

Forensic Psychiatry is the application of the principles of general psychiatry to those mentally disordered patients who have offended, or are likely to offend, or for management reasons have been or remain subject to detention either in a health facility or in prison. The curriculum proffered the following definition for forensic psychiatric nursing, 'the employment of psychiatric nursing skills to address the needs of mentally disordered patients who have offended, or are likely to offend, or are subject to detention within the terms of legislation.

The outline curriculum deliberately avoided the inclusion of acquiring experience in physical intervention skills, forming a part of the course. Instead, it was expected that emphasis would be placed on the examination of ethical, moral and legal issues pertinent to physical restraint along with practice in incident analysis. Course members would, however, have an opportunity to examine current courses in control and restraint as regards suitability for staff. This specialist panel responsible for providing the outline curriculum were of the opinion that the training of staff in physical intervention skills was an employers responsibility to all staff who needed to care for difficult patients and that such training should be available as part of a planned introduction to the expected responsibilities of the duties to be performed.

The purpose of the course was to provide the opportunity for registered nurses to participate in clearly structured and negotiated educational experiences which would enable them to work more effectively as nurse practitioners in a multi-professional setting, providing nursing care within a controlled environment. The course intended to provide for theoretical studies and planned associated experience for nurses contemplating working, or already working, in controlled environments.

The course was expected to be in two stages, the first stage comprising of a modular approach looking at;

- Foundation material on professional practice, common to all courses at post basic level according to local agreements on common core curriculum.

- Subject material related to the principles of psychiatric nursing in controlled environments. This stage was expected to mimic in large parts the ENB 960 course which was its fore- runner.

Stage two was expected to build on material covered in stage one and provide specialist modules leading to the award of the certificate issued by the National Board. The specialist modules would contain topics and planned experiences specific to the field under study and acknowledge the requirements of individual course members as regards their area of work on the basis of negotiated curriculum. Stage one was a pre-requisite to commencing the certificated stage two part of the course. Evidence of previous educational experience would enable course applicants to negotiate exemptions from certain parts of the course. The broad aims of the course were;

- To develop and adapt present skills and acquire new skills in meeting the needs of people who are mentally disordered and receiving care within a controlled environment.

- To acquire and extend the essential knowledge base within the specific field of practice.

- To examine course members own attitudes and develop a positive approach towards mentally disordered people.

- To facilitate a greater awareness of the nurse practitioner responsibility for the nursing component of care within the plan of treatment agreed by the multi-professional team.

In achieving the above aim educational experiences would be provided to:

- Assist the course members to identify individual educational needs.

- Encourage the course members to undertake responsibility for their own learning through individual negotiated educational experiences.

- Enable course members to acquire a sound knowledge base linked to the skills component of the course.

- Explore the variety of nursing skills and provide opportunities to practice.

- Influence the development of appropriate attitudes.

The entry requirements for the above course permitted registered nurse whose names appeared on part three (RMN) or part five (RNMH) of the professional register of the United Kingdom Central Council for Nursing, Midwifery and Health Visiting. Successful completion of the course leads to the award of a certificate of competence issued by the Board.

The first course venue to be approved by the National Board to run ENB CNS 770 'Nursing in Controlled Environments' was the post basic and continuing education department at Ashworth Hospital, Merseyside. Mr Paul Tarbuck, Director of Advanced Nursing Studies at Ashworth Hospital is to be applauded for this significant milestone in the history of Forensic Psychiatric Nursing. He strived from the mid 80's, formally as a ENB specialist panel member for the generation of the outline curriculum for the course 770 and subsequently as a member of the Department of Health Specialist Panel on Forensic Nursing. The first course of its kind commenced in October 1990 and without the dedicated efforts of Mr Tarbuck together with the energies of this books editors, this collective piece of work concerning aspects of forensic psychiatric nursing would never have materialised.

In generating the curriculum contents for the Ashworth course the curriculum planning team assumed that the following would underpin all its deliberations:

- A person is a sentient being with unique features that characterise the individual and set him/her apart from other individuals. Persons are, in the main, gregarious, actively seeking the companionship of others. In life, a person constantly affects and is affected by the human and material environment in which he/she exists. Human beings have fundamental rights to freedom of will; autonomy; informed consent; consultation and appropriate health care when and where needed, and that rights should be limited only if the exercising of rights involves unnecessarily compromising personal security needs, and/or failing to take reasonable account of the security needs of others.

- Human beings exist in societies arranged to allow association and for mutual benefit and common interest. This may be accompanied by harmonisation of the individuals' values, beliefs, customs and the creating of laws, so that societies themselves develop unique characteristics and cultural attributes.

- Health is a state of optimum functioning in the whole individual as an integrated entity. Illness is a state of non-optimum functioning in a part, or the whole of the body. Permanent forms of illness are disabilities of optimum functioning.

- Nursing is an activity licensed by society concerning assessing, planning, implementing and evaluating strategies of care designed to assist individuals to return to a state of health, or to assist with an acceptable adjustment to a state of disability or loss. The process of nursing cannot be divorced from the interpersonal nature of human existence.

- Psychiatric nursing is concerned with advocating mental health, arresting and limiting psychological disorders, and with assisting human beings in mental health endeavours (Antonovsky Josse-Bass, 1979).

Nursing in controlled environments is the employment of those skills necessary to address the needs of the ill individual who have offended, or is likely to offend, or who remains subject to detention within the terms of legislation (ENB, 1988). I am of the opinion that the above assumptions should form an integral part of any philosophy of care to be found within controlled environments and should, wherever possible, be embraced by the charter of patients rights to be found within the same environment.

Forensic behavioural science

The University of Liverpool have recently commenced a two year, part-time course leading to the degree of Master of Science in Forensic Behavioural Science. The first year intends to follow a prearranged curriculum and on successful completion of it students can elect to be awarded a diploma in Forensic Behavioural Science. For the award of the Masters Degree, students will be required to complete a second year consisting largely of the conduct of a research project and preparation of a thesis. The course is based in the sub department of clinical psychology within the department of psychiatry. However, it is intended to be multi-disciplinary in content and orientation and parts of the teaching will be undertaken by members of other University departments and by external lecturers.

Rationale

There is no single word which encompasses the entire spectrum of legal, mental health, or social services which operate within the United Kingdom, but one thing can be said about it that is surely beyond dispute. In its scale, in the numbers and types of persons who work within it, in the nature of its decisions and in the rules that govern them, it represents a creature of awesome complexity. The system of police, courts, and penal institutions is bewildering enough on its own; that of clinics, hospitals, and allied health services equally if not more so; while a range of other social services and of the statutory or voluntary, national or local agencies who deliver them, seems beyond the capacity of most citizens to grasp. To have to deal with any one sector of this panoply of officialdom is a forbidding enough prospect in itself. To be enmeshed in the intricacies that result when two or more agencies are involved is more perplexing still. For those on whom decisions have to be made by a variety of agencies occupying different positions in the system, the result can be a state of complete incomprehension. Unfortunately, this is often paralleled by a similar state of confusion amongst the personnel who inhabit different work places inside the system (Glasgow, McGuire, 1989). The course arose out of a concern that the complexities of the system are such that it often fails to deliver services adequately, or to achieve its own stated goals. Communication between its constituent parts can often be faulty, linguistic and conceptual barriers can inhibit a genuine discussion of ideas and messages are not conveyed. The risks of this may be greatest of all for individuals, processed simultaneously by legal, health, and social services departments, from mentally disordered offenders to children alleged to have been abused, families, communities or victims affected by any decisions that are made about them.

The basic purpose of the course is to gather together a group of students from a variety of professional backgrounds and expose them to a mixture of teaching spread across all of the disciplines whom they represent. By examining each others views, exchanging their experiences and being provided with a course designed to stimulate real multi-professional discussion, they might develop an integrated view of how the above mentioned 'system' actually works.

The initially stated aim of the course, which lead to its establishment and which has been the central idea in guiding the development of the syllabus, is; to equip practitioners at the meeting point of the legal, clinical and social services professions with the specialised knowledge and skills they need to become more effective in their work.

Sixteen course members were recruited and I understand they have just completed the first year/diploma level of the course. They were drawn, as expected, from a wide range of professions, including nursing, probation, police and prison services, social work and psychology. Of the fifteen course members, seven are currently practising nurses with or without involvement at Senior Management level. The nursing profession should soon enjoy the fruits of their labours in the form of publications that will assist in the identification of the skills and knowledge base required of nurses working at the interface between the criminal justice system, Health and Social Services.

Special Hospital Service Authority

The Special Hospital Service Authority took over the running of the Special Hospitals Service on the 1 October 1989. The immediate task of the authority was to get a firm grip on its management responsibilities whilst at the same time launching initiatives which would help shape the strategy for the medium to long term by testing fresh approaches to care and providing new information. At the time that the SHSA was set up, the Government gave them the following set of six overall objectives:

- To ensure the continuing safety of the public.

- To ensure the provision of appropriate treatment for patients.

- Ensure a good quality of life for patients and staff.

- Develop the hospitals as centres of excellence for the training of staff in all disciplines in forensic and other branches of psychiatry and psychiatric care and treatment.

- Develop closer working relationships with NHS local and regional psychiatric services.

- To promote research in fields related to forensic psychiatry.

From the outset, the authority has been committed to the six objectives outlined above. Central to the above objectives, has been the commitment to focus upon the need to provide the best quality of care and treatment for their patients. Charles Kay, Chief Executive of the SHSA, said in the introduction to the SHSA review 1991 'the real justification for any health authorities existence must rest on what it achieves for its patients. The well meaning endeavour from the centre will be hollow if it cannot be related to the conditions of caring and the success of treatment' (SHSA, 1991).

The SHSA development plan of 1991-96 contains five major themes, these are;

- To engage in joint action with other agencies in the long term interests of patients.

- To obtain a better balance between quality and security of care.

- To remain open to the views and influences of others.

- To promote staff development and change the culture of the hospitals.

- To manage the business.

The SHSA is committed towards the pursuit of the principle aim of providing the necessary framework to achieve the changes which would lead to the highest possible standards of care and treatment for its patients. They considered that the achievement of such aims would be dependent on changing in the culture within each of the three Special Hospitals. They strongly believe that the basis of cultural change lies in the devolution of responsibility and ensuring that decisions in relation to patient care are taken at the point nearest to, and in partnership with, the patient.

As part of this process the SHSA published its strategy for nursing 'Nursing in Special Hospitals' in November 1991. Now, for the first time, nurses in Special Hospitals have a strategic framework for the future, designed to build on past success and to clearly set the way for the future development of this very important and challenging branch of psychiatric nursing. The strategy for nursing describes how the objectives of the SHSA will be translated into nursing practise and champions the therapeutic role of its nursing staff within what is a very unique nursing situation. The SHSA are committed towards ensuring that each and every nurse within the hospitals has the best possible support, training and direction to enable them to provide an improved quality of care for their patients. Personally, I am left in no doubt whatsoever that, in future years, the Special Hospitals will be a very exciting place indeed to practise forensic psychiatric nursing skills.

'Nursing in Special Hospitals' is intended to communicate to staff both within and outside the authority, the aspirations of the nursing workforce in what it is setting out to achieve over coming years. Frank Powell, Head of Nursing Services within the SHSA believes the above aspirations 'belong not to the Special Hospitals but to every individual nurse working with them. Each persons endeavour to achieve their contribution to the fulfilment of them will make the Special Hospitals a service that nurses can be proud to work in and be part of'.

The key aim within the nursing strategy most likely to achieve an enhanced quality of care for patients is the integration of the education of all nurses with their clinical practice. This will require that the clinical practice area, rather than the classroom needs to be perceived as the environment within which continuing education and in-service training for nurses takes place. This will require both managers and practitioners to have an equal part to play in education and training facilitated by nurse educators.

Nursing education has a well established base within the 'Ashworth Centre' and many aspects of activities within this centre is distinctly multi-disciplinary. The centre provides induction and in-service training programmes as well as continuing and advanced nursing education. Basic nursing courses are now provided by Edge Hill College of Further Education in conjunction with Sefton Health Authority and are no longer the direct responsibility of teachers at Ashworth Hospital. In December 1991, Paul Tarbuck was appointed as Director of Advanced

Nursing Studies at the centre and he is establishing strong links between his tutorial staff and the five newly appointed Clinical Area Nurse Managers within the Special Hospital. This link is intended to promote the aim of integration of education and practice and emphasis will be placed upon educational programmes responding to clinical requirements. This, of course, will require each nurse to share responsibility for their own personal development.

The SHSA is actively engaged in bringing about change - change which is necessary to improve the care and treatment of its patients and to involve them in that process. Nurses form the major workforce within the Special Hospitals and although sensational newspaper headlines have concentrated upon highlighting failure within the hospitals, it is necessary to remember that a great deal of quality nursing takes place and the positive plans for the future, who's foundations have already been laid, will achieve the changes to which everyone is committed. It is relatively easy to criticise (the SHSA are sometimes harsh on themselves) but it is much harder for people to commit themselves to a process of change which is lengthy and arduous. Many good staff work within the Special Hospitals and are committed to the goal of creating an excellent service, they believe it can be achieved, all forensic psychiatric nurses (and other nurses for that matter) have a duty to assist in achieving this goal.

Diversion from custody

In September 1990 the Home Office issued a circular (HC66/90) entitled 'Provision for Mentally Disordered Offenders'. The purpose of the circular was to draw the attention of the courts and those services responsible for dealing with mentally disordered persons who commit, or are suspected of committing, criminal offences to:

- The legal powers which exist.

- The desirability of ensuring effective co-operation between agencies to ensure that the best use is made of resources and that mentally disordered persons are not prosecuted where this is not required by the public interest.

Government policy requires that, wherever possible, mentally disordered persons should receive care and treatment from the Health and Social Services. Where there is sufficient evidence, in accordance with the principles of the Code for Crown Prosecutors, the show that a mentally disordered person has committed an offence, careful consideration should be given to whether prosecution is required in the public interest. It is desirable that alternatives to prosecution, such as cautioning by the police, and/or admission to hospital, if the persons mental condition requires hospital treatment or support in the community, should be considered first before deciding that prosecution is necessary. The Government recognises that this policy can only be effective if the courts and criminal justice agencies have access to health and social services. This will require consultation and co-operation, and this circular aims to provide guidance on the establishment of the satisfactory working relationship between the agencies concerned (Home Office, 1990).

Unfortunately, users find the title of this health circular, somewhat misleading. The title implies that any person being considered for diversion from the criminal justice system to the health and social services has committed an offence. Yet this clearly is not the case, the whole document (HC66/90) targets persons who have not committed an offence, those who are suspected of having committed an offence, those who have committed an offence (and might subsequently be prosecuted) and those persons who have committed an offence but it is not considered necessary in the publics interest to arrest that person for the offence.

Having established that the circular applies generally to mentally disordered persons and not just to mentally disordered offenders then it becomes clearer that diversion, as a general rule, should be sought within a placement that is within the least restrictive setting possible appropriate to the patients clinical condition and subject to the absolute need to ensure the safety of the patient, health care staff and to the public. The treatment and care available to all psychiatric patients, including mentally disordered offenders or potential offenders, should be based on the same clinical principles and professional procedures.

It is the need for any degree of security required to enable treatment to be provided effectively and safely which, to a large extent, determines the facility in which the patient should be accommodated.

I think it important, from the outset of planning of district services in accordance with the guidance in circular 66/90, to emphasise that forensic psychiatric services, as a tertiary service, must not seek to in any way undermine or presume upon the relationship which should properly be developed between the general psychiatric services and the criminal justice system.

What remains to be seen is whether or not commitment is forthcoming from general psychiatry services in demonstrating their willingness to extend such services towards, the police stations, courts and prisons, and to compliment these commitments I see no reason why nominated community psychiatric nurses should not offer their services to both the courts and police stations along lines described in annexe b, paragraph 10 and annexe c, paragraph 2 of the circular.

People with mental disorders who commit offences come into contact with a wide range of different agencies and appear at various junctures within the criminal justice system. National and local experience shows that this leads to an uncoordinated approach. No single agency assumes clear responsibility for a case, often resulting in the inappropriate placement of a mentally disordered person in the prison either on remand or to serve a sentence. There are a number of schemes operational at the moment, one of which is the Hertfordshire psychiatric assessment panel scheme which was initiated to provide a forum for an inter-agency approach for each offender February 1991 saw the launch of the 'Birmingham Court Liaison Project', an inter-agency project at the Victoria Law Courts in Birmingham designed to bring about the diversion of offenders from the court system. The project, which seeks to put into practice the philosophy enshrined in Home Office circular 66/90, brings together representatives of the West Midlands probation service, West Midlands police, the courts and the NHS. Instrumental within this multi-agency initiative is the involvement of community forensic psychiatric nurses and medical practitioners from the Reaside Clinic in Rubery, Birmingham. Community psychiatric nurses from the Clinic have been assigned to help identify mentally disordered offenders held overnight in police cells following arrest. Each morning, a CPN makes an initial assessment after reviewing the necessary papers and interviewing those defendants whose condition and background suggest a possible mental disorder. A Senior Registrar in forensic psychiatry from the Reaside

Clinic may, if required, be called in subsequently to confirm the diagnosis and liaise with local psychiatric services. In cases where compulsory admission to a psychiatric hospital is indicated, a second medical practitioner from a general psychiatric hospital and an approved social worker are invited to help assess the patient and sign the necessary papers. Following the assessment stage, court officers are notified whether psychiatric treatment is require. The Crown Prosecution Service then decides whether the matter should be discontinued.

This scheme is proving to be very cost effective and during the first six months of the scheme, a total of 203 defendants awaiting their first court appearance were assessed by the CPN's. Mental disorder was detected or suspected in 109 cases. Of these:

- 33 were referred for in-patient assessment and treatment in general psychiatric hospitals;

- 49 received out-patient assessment and treatment at general psychiatric hospitals;

- 3 were referred to a Regional Secure Unit;

- 15 received out-patient assessment and treatment from the forensic psychiatry service;

- 9 were remanded in custody.

Overall, the scheme is considered successful and has received favourable comment from the Reed Committee. On 6 January 1992 it was, in fact, extended to Coventry and will start up in Wolverhampton in April of the same year. Inspector Colin Murphy of West Midlands Police believes that there may be scope for extending the scheme. 'In an ideal world the involvement of the CPN's would extend to the point where they would be sent to the police station before a decision is taken about a charge, or that decision would be deferred pending an assessment being made'. That point of view is one shared by Reaside's Director of Nursing and Operational Services and Chairman of the

Forensic Psychiatric Nurses Association, Mr Tony Hillis. 'At present the police station calls out the police surgeon. I would suspect that CPN's, because of their knowledge and contacts, might be able to divert more appropriately from a police station than some police surgeons' (Nursing Times, 1991). There is a great need for this valuable service to be re-provided in localities throughout the rest of the United Kingdom.

Nursing leaders as product champions

This chapter would be incomplete if I overlooked such a vital opportunity to celebrate the 'product champions' of forensic psychiatric nursing. In wishing to celebrate the individual contributions made towards the development of services for mentally disordered offenders I was conscious of my personal bias towards the RSU programme and therefore I sought the opinion of colleagues from wide and far who were representative of the whole movement. Of course, each of them have had personal experiences which have exposed them, in varying degrees, to innovative leaders. But, I am comforted by the knowledge that there exists a consensus of opinion across the United Kingdom as to the worth of the following contributions and their significance. Mr John Tait and Mr Tony Backer-Holst were applauded for the manner in which they were seen to be supportive towards the development of a national regional secure unit programme. Chief Nursing Officers working within the Special Hospitals were singled out for special attention, Alan Lee commissioned a new Special Hospital (Park Lane) with a vision different from his former colleagues within the older establishment. Marion Hendry introduced openness to the Special Hospital at Rampton with her charismatic leadership skills being used effectively to bring about change. The new breed of nurse managers within the Special Hospitals are energetically involved in taking this sterling work further.

The grandfather of the RSU programme, Mr John Parry has been extremely influential in the development of forensic psychiatric nursing. His words of wisdom, presentation and style have encouraged and persuaded many of the non-believers. He commissioned the first interim secure unit of its kind back in 1976 at Rainhill Hospital in

Merseyside, subsequently developed, commissioned and made operational a purpose built 50 bedded Regional Secure Unit called the Scott Clinic and has since managed the service with grim determination and an abundance of skill. He promoted the early conferences at Padgate and Chester which emphasised the need for multi-disciplinary team working. The mix of different disciplines attending those conferences was amazing and it proved to be a trend setter within the discipline of forensic psychiatry. The conferences achieved a togetherness which promoted commitment and ownership of an extremely difficult problem. He, more than anyone else has promoted the principle of community based services for mentally disordered offenders and has been supported in this drive towards community care by Dave Baylis, one of the first Forensic CPN's recognised as a product champion of community care for mentally disordered offenders. Clinical care within the Scott Clinic has been enhanced tremendously by the quiet, realistic enthusiasm of John Kilshaw who's contribution to 'caring' has been immense. Mr Parry is currently a member of the 'Reed Committee' and I am sure he will be able to apply his wealth of knowledge to the problems faced by this committee in meeting the future challenge.

Mr Parry has demonstrated his many abilities in managing the Merseyside Regional Secure Unit programme of developments through to fruition, he encountered terrific opposition from the trade unions in previous years, cultural difficulties were courted from the parent hospital but despite this he continues to impose a deeply caring influence upon the services.

On the educational and research front, Cliff Johnson from the English National Board has, for a long time now, recognised the educational needs of nurses working within these challenging environments and has facilitated the passage of new initiatives in nurse education for forensic psychiatric nurses. Each of the Special Hospitals has its own product champion in the 'research arena'. Robinson in Rampton Hospital, Burrows in Broadmoor Hospital and Mason in Ashworth have all contributed material subsequently published in the Nursing Press and are currently engaged in research of specific relevance to the specialty of forensic psychiatric nursing. In the West Midlands Tony Hillis brought rich values and philosophies down to service delivery level. He has made a major contribution to the development of services for mentally disordered offenders by paying specific attention to detail in recruiting nurses to this specialty. The quality of staff is of paramount importance and he recognised the need for the service to avoid the 'machismo' and those staff with controlling inclinations. Never before had attention been paid to staff profiling so as to ensure that the client remained at the centre of all our caring endeavours. He, more than anyone else has demonstrated that realistic alternatives to seclusion do in fact exist.

2 The clinical nurse specialist in forensic settings

Richard Benson

The clinical grading structure has focused attention on those nurses who hold a Clinical Nurse Specialist (CNS) title. As in other areas of nursing CNS's are increasingly being employed in Regional Secure Units (RSU's). There appears to be no published work on the role of the CNS working in a RSU and it therefore remains unclear what the specialist nature of a Forensic Clinical Nurse Specialist (FCNS) is, as opposed to a CNS working in generic psychiatry. Parry (1991) and Pederson (1988) described forensic psychiatric nursing as a speciality because of the unique relationship between crime and mental illness and also because of the secure nature of RSU's. The question of whether specific skills and knowledge are required in order to work with mentally disordered patients in secure environments remains unanswered.

Niskala (1988) attempted to identify the essential components of nurse's work in Canadian in forensic settings. Of the thirteen components she identified only two: maintaining security and instructing offenders were the components that could be described as being unique to forensic psychiatric nurses. Merely being involved in a narrow range of activity does not in itself warrant the title 'specialist'.

In a small study that is described in this chapter, an attempt was made to explore the knowledge and skills of some nurses working in forensic units in the UK. The study involved the use of the repertory

45

grid technique to explore how a small group of forensic nurses and clinical nurse specialists viewed their roles.

Clinical specialisation in forensic care

Clinical specialisation was first reported by DeWitt (1900) who described specialist areas of nursing practice. Peplau (1965) described the development of specialisation in nursing as originating from the move by progressive nurses towards areas which particularly interested them, and in which the opportunity to specialise existed. As these nurses both trained and had further clinical experience in the specialist areas they were regarded as clinical experts. Stafford (1991) suggests that the role of the Clinical Nurse Specialist (CNS) first emerged as a result of the part played by the U.S. Mobile Army Surgical Hospitals (MASH) during warfare. During the Second World War and the Korean and Vietnam Wars, nurses were responsible for delivering a sophisticated level of care to those suffering from severe mental and physical conditions.

The American nursing literature relating to the CNS in the 1960's and 70's showed confusion in the profession regarding the preparation, functions, responsibilities and placement of the CNS in the bureaucratic structure (Hamric 1983, Ropka and Kay 1984). Much of this work focused on justifying the need for masters degree prepared nurses to remain involved in direct patient care, and in developing a label for this new role. Mallison (1984) suggested that by the late 1960's and early 1970's, it was becoming accepted that progression within the profession should not always necessitate a move away from direct patient care.

Definitions of the CNS role were formulated in both the United States (Ropka and Fry 1984) and in Canada (Registered Nurses Association of Ontario 1976). Callaghan (1990) argued that the Briggs (1972) recommendation for a career in clinical nursing for Senior Nurses led to a call for the introduction of roles such as that of the CNS in the U.K.

Christman (1965) pointed out that the name or title of this new specialist was less important than the implications of specialisation for the nursing profession. He felt that through specialisation, nursing practice could be constantly refined and could keep abreast of new knowledge. The literature suggests that the role of the CNS encompasses more than the need to be an expert practitioner in a chosen field and points to a multi-purpose role for the CNS. Castledine (1982) defined the CNS as a:

Trained nurse with additional nursing education, who has been carrying out direct clinical nursing practice with specific patients in a special branch of nursing.

Castledine (1983) went on to identify eleven key factors relating to the role of the CNS. The National League for Nursing (1958) put forward a definition of the CNS in psychiatric nursing as:

Bringing about advances in the art and science of psychiatric nursing and promoting the application of new knowledge and methods in the care of patients.

Although this acknowledges the role of the CNS in promoting progressive practices, it fails to explain how this promotion can be achieved. Callaghan (1990) put forward the multi-faceted role of the CNS at the Maudsley Hospital and described them as an:

Expert practitioner with considerable experience and additional nursing education and/or education in a related discipline whose function is to advance the practice of psychiatric nursing and act as a consultant to nursing and other health care personnel, an educator, research resource person and manager.

The Clinical Nurse Advisory Group at the Maudsley Hospital proposed a common core group job description for CNS's, encompassing all of the above duties. Throughout the published material on the role of the CNS, the components that appear to be cited most often are those of practitioner, educator, consultant, researcher and change agent (Fenton 1985, Storr 1988, Ropka and Fay 1984, Fife and Hemler 1983).

The role of the clinical nurse specialist

Practitioner

The advanced preparation of the CNS should enable them to deal with unusual problems. There should be more emphasis on greater deliberation and use of reason than would be expected of a generically trained, staff nurse (Calkin 1984). Fenton (1985) suggested that as a result of understanding the experience of patients and their families coming into hospital, the CNS can act as a patient advocate.

Tarsitano et al (1980) found that neither CNS's nor administrators considered routine patient care as a role of the CNS. In support of this argument Metcalfe et al (1984) point out that by being involved in direct patient care the effectiveness of the CNS may be reduced as they would be less able to facilitate the developmental needs of other staff members. Kerrane (1975) in summarising the responsibilities of CNS's in the USA, specifically identified direct patient care as a major component of the CNS's role. The CNS Advisory Group at the Maudsley Hospital felt it to be the job of the CNS to assess, plan and implement those aspects of care to the patients and their families that required their specialist skills and knowledge.

What seems to be unclear from this brief review of the CNS's role is whether or not he or she should focus primarily on patient care or should emphasise, further, his or her role as staff developer and trainer. This point is developed in the next section.

Educator

The CNS's role as educator involves health teaching within a nursing framework for both patients and their families and other care staff. The education component with nursing staff also entails developing the other nurse's teaching skills (Metcalfe et al 1984, Kerrane 1975). Dierschel (1976) stated that the CNS can be a valuable resource for information and guidance because their background and job flexibility enables them to carry out literature searches that other nurses may not have the time or skills to do. Fife and Humber (1983) suggested that a valuable arena for the CNS to use her educating role is the ward round, where existing problems and needs can be discussed. It would follow from this suggestion that nursing team meetings would be suitable forums for the CNS to practice teaching.

Consultant

Barron (1983) claimed that the value of the nurse acting as consultants to other nurses outside their immediate environment is a relatively new concept. Barron explained that if a truly consultative role is adopted, the consultee should both initiate the process and also be able to accept or reject the consultant's recommendations. Therefore, those CNS's with management responsibilities whose recommendations are not easily rejected by ward based staff are not real 'consultants'. A possible benefit of using the CNS as a consultant is their ability not only to assist staff with assessment, but also to facilitate a holistic perspective by enabling nurses to examine their own perceptions, feelings and behaviours, as well as those of patients and their families (Fife and Humber 1983). If a CNS is to act as a consultant for other staff involved in care, there is the prospect of overlaping or possibly, contradicting the work of other health care professionals (Barron 1983). It would therefore seem important for the CNS to be assured of support from their manager and for the CNS to have the skills to negotiate boundaries with other professionals.

Researcher

The research role of the CNS is heavily supported in many of published works, (Kerrane 1975, Castledine 1983, Stafford 1991, Callaghan 1990). However, it is one that has not easily been translated into practice. Tarsitano et al (1980) found a large discrepancy in the perceived importance of research to the CNS between administrators and CNS's, with the administrators rating it as more important than the CNS's did. Storr (1988) suggests that this may be accounted for by the difficulties CNS's have in conducting research. These difficulties include time constraints, lack of funding, a lack of CNS role models who have succeeded in this task. Another constraint may be the lack of education and training that is available to CNS's in the field of research methods leading to a skills deficit in the CNS's.

49

Hodgeman (1983) in reviewing the published work on the research role stated that the CNS 'seemed to be the repository of all the professionals, hitherto unfulfilled hopes and dreams'. It was envisaged that the CNS would generate clinical nursing research. Castledine (1983) found that few CNS's had the education to enable them to evaluate or carry out nursing research. Hodgson (1983) suggested that the CNS should be able to interpret research findings and serve as a role model who makes use of research to solve nursing problems. Until CNSs have sufficient educational background, they will remain unable to fulfil these much needed requirements. Their ability to conduct and utilise research findings in clinical settings remains untapped.

Change agent

Everson (1981) pointed out that there is widespread support for the expectation of the CNS to act as a catalyst for widespread change in clinical settings. If CNS's are not in a managerial postion, they may not have the power to effect change, directly. If they are in managerial posts they can exert their positional power to assist in bringing about change (Everson 1981). On the other hand, the coercive use of power in trying to effect change may not be the most effective method.

CNS's, as relative 'outisders' may not perceive themselves to be powerful change agents. This may be because management in health service systems has tended to be hierarchical, with power be exerted by those higher up the management hierarchy. If CNS's are viewed as consultants and as standing slightly outside of that traditional hierarchy, then they may find traditional power-coercive forms of change difficult to effect. There may, however, be plenty of scope, here, for a more democratic means of effective change. Negotiation, discussion and consensus, may all have their part to play in this sort of change process. One thing seems clear: if CNS's are to be change agents, they will have to work closely with both managers and clinical nurses.

Staff advocate

Another function of the CNS that is beginning to appear in the literature is that of staff advocate. Fife and Lember (1983) indicate that the CNS can assist staff with the prevention and resolution of conflicts and thereby decrease their levels of stress and increase their levels of clinical functioning. A survey by Melcalfe et al (1984) noted that the CNS is often used by staff for counselling and guidance. Storr (1988) suggests that the reason for these activities becoming part of the CNS's role is their constant visibility and obvious commitment to a high quality of patient care.

Other issues

A Royal College of Nursing (RCN) working party examining the role of nursing specialities and specialist nursing roles (RCN 1988). It stated that specialist practice involved a clinical and consultative role, a teaching role, a management role and the application of relevant research. The working party went on to state that only if a nurse was involved in all four of these practices could they call themselves a CNS. If this really is the case, then the CNS is being asked to do a great deal. It is possible to question whether or not this is a realistic appraisal of the role of the CNS.

Castledine (1983) identified eleven key elements of the role of the CNS. He then surveyed a group of over 300 nurses identified as Clinical Nurse Specialists. His findings suggested that although some nurses came close to fulfilling the criteria, not one of those surveyed fulfilled it completely.

Casteldine suggested that several common factors contributed to this result. Few of his sample held higher academic qualifications and only 2 out of the 300 surveyed held a masters degree in nursing. Moreover, only a small number of people had work published relating to their specialist field and few were able to evaluate or carry out nursing research. A majority of nurses did not accept the exercising of accountability as an important or significant factor in their job and many were tied to the traditional nursing hierarchy, therefore not allowing themselves the freedom and flexibility to act independently. Although many of those surveyed were competent at clinical nursing assessment, few could prove they were experts in using the nursing process approach.

A exploratory study

The study described here was intended to examine the roles and functions of CNS's and to compare the self-perceptions of forensic and generic CNS's. It was envisaged that certain skills and knowledge specific to forensic psychiatric nursing would be identified.

Sample

A convenience sample of ten CNS's was interviewed. Five of the sample were based at regional secure units and five worked in general psychiatry.

Methodology

In order to look at the different skills and knowledge of forensic CNS's and CNS's a structured interview technique was used based on a Repertory Grid Technique (Kelly 1955). The grid technique is a flexible and economical data gathering device and may be used to systematically explore and record a person's views during interviews (Fransella and Bannister, 1977). In order to get an individual to share his views a knowledge about the important 'elements' and 'constructs' held by each individual, is required. An element may be any object, event or person which the person is asked to consider. Typically, a set of elements is chosen by the researcher and the interviewee is asked to identify important 'likenesses' and important 'differences' between two or three of these at any one time. This procedure usually generates a set of bi-polar constructs, for example, good-bad, cruel-kind and so on. A construct is a dimension or characteristic which has two poles, and provides a basis for understanding how people perceive a number of elements. The grid procedure allows the researcher to examine how the elements and constructs are interrelated.

Applications of grid technique in nursing research

Although PCT and the grid technique is grounded in the clinical field there have been surprisingly few research studies using the method in the field of nursing. However, a small number of studies have been reported, which used the method to good effect, but these have tended to emphasise the quantitative characteristics of the grid technique following in the footsteps of many psychological applications.

Wilkinson (1982), used the grid technique to examine the effects of a psychiatric allocation on general nursing students attitudes to psychiatric patients, while Davis (1983) explored a range of aspects of student nurse training. In addition, Heyman et. al. (1983) studied the socialization process of nursing trainees in British hospitals using personal construct theory, and Costigan et. al. (1987) investigated nurses' perceptions of attempted suicide. Recently, Pollock (1987) has used the technique in her exploration of the role of the community psychiatric nurse. Notably few research studies using the grid technique have been completed in different areas of nursing, despite successful psychological applications in clinical and educational settings (Beail, 1985), and in the realm of management and commerce (Stewart and Stewart, 1981).

A notable feature of most of these investigations in the field of nursing is their use of quite large samples, and a reliance on sophisticated statistical analysis to interpret the grid data. While such applications are perfectly legitimate and feasible they do require that the researcher has access to computing facilities, and stress the quantitative facets of grid analysis.

However, it is also possible to use the grid with limited resources to produce important insights and understandings, by examining both qualitative and quantitative information contained in the grid.

Procedure

Two workshops were set up, one looking at forensic skills and knowledge, the other at general psychiatric nursing skills. The first workshop comprised psychiatric nurses, all of at least charge nurse grade, who were working in forensic environments. The second workshop consisted of similar grades of psychiatric nurses who had recently been working in general psychiatry settings. Both sets of workshops participants were presented with a list of thirty three elements which were a collection of the subjects that formed the basis of the Ashworth Hospital ENB 770 course curriculum. Although the course is forensic in nature it appeared possible to identify within it, elements that were applicable to all aspects of psychiatric nursing.

During both workshops, participants were asked to identify the six elements of skill and knowledge that were most pertinent to the role of the CNS in their own area of work. As well as the thirty three elements provided, the workshop participants were advised that they could add any other elements that they felt to be important. Six key elements were identified within each of the workshops and those elements are illustrated in figure 2.1

Clinical nurse specialists	Forensic clinical nurse specialists
1. Staff management	1. Assessment and management of dangerous behaviours
2. Teaching	2. Criminology
3. Research	3. Law and professional accountability
4. Self-awareness	4. Therapeutic use of security
5. Management of care	5. Social policy
6. Interpersonal skills	6. Ethics

Figure 2.1 Workshop results

Following the collection of these data a group of ten clinical nurse specialists, both forensic and general, were invited to explore the twelve elements using a modified version of the repertory grid approach to structure the conversation. The following paragraphs identify some of the issues that emerged from that discussion.

Staff management

All the CNS's, considered the management of staff to be of importance to their job, and a majority were involved with it frequently or very frequently. This emphasis placed on the management role falls in line with a recommendation of the RCN working party (1988), which states that CNS's as leading practitioners should have management power in order in influence practice. This view is shared by Hanrick and Spross (1983) who emphasised the need for CNS's to have legitimate power and authority and that they should not only be expert in providing direct patient care, but also in controlling and coordinating care staff. In order to achieve this proposed level of expertise a substantial background of formal training in management might be expected, however, only four of the informants claimed to have high degree of formal training. Thus, although most of the informants felt that staff management was an important part of their role, few of them felt formally prepared for the task.

Assessing and managing dangerous behaviours

There was some difference of opinion about assessing and managing dangerous behaviour in clinical settings. While the forensic respondents felt it was a particularly important part of their role, fewer of the general clinical nurse specialists felt that it was part of their role. Two of the general specialists felt that it was of very little importance in their daily work. This seems to point to a role difference that might be explored further.

Most of the forensic respondents were frequently involved in the management and assessment of dangerous behaviour. Only occasionally were general respondents involved in this sort of assessment. Two of the forensic respondents claimed to be either expert or very competent in this facet of their work. Again, more work needs to be done to clarify both how dangerousness might be assessed and also how nurses might be trained to do this.

None of the forensic respondents claimed to have formal training in this domain but a number suggested that they had received some instruction in this area. The general respondents said they had very little formal training and instruction in this area of work.

Castledine (1983) suggested that a nurse must have significant formal training in their specialist area in order to call themselves a clinical nurse specialist. It follows that if the assessment and management of dangerous behaviours is to be considered as a major component of the specialist nature of forensic psychiatric nursing, then FCNS's should have a recognised level of training in it. This absence of formal training may be attributed to the lack of relevant courses available, which in raises the question of whether or not nurses do have a unique knowledge of the assessment and management of dangerous behaviours.

Teaching

All respondents felt that teaching was an important aspect of their role and six felt that they were quite skilled in this facet of the job. Few, though, have any formal training in teaching. This also open two questions: whether or not clinical nurse specialists can be called specialists in Castledine's sense of the term and whether or not appropriate facilities exist for the formal training of such practitioners.

Interpersonal skills

All respondents felt that effective interpersonal skills were the basis of good practice. However, while four of the general respondents considered themselves to be interpersonally competent, only two of the forensic respondents made such a claim. Also, four of the general respondents said that they had received significant training in this area whilst only one of the forensic respondents had. It is notable that the idea of competence in the interpersonal field is a relatively new one in psychiatric nurse training and can be traced back to the introduction of a revised syllabus of training for psychiatric nurses that was first published in 1982. It is possible that in forensic psychiatry, the emphasis is more on containment than on therapeutic relationships and this may be a factor in some forensic nurses feeling less interpersonally competent than their general counterparts.

Management of care

In accordance with the emphasis given to the Clinical Management role of the CNS, by the RCN working party (1988). There appears to be no significant differences in the role of CNS and FCNS in this area.

The law and professional accountability

There was no important difference in the ratings given by either set of CNS's with both scoring highly for importance, competency and frequency. Law and professional accountability were perceived by the respondents to be important and issues which effect daily practice. Also, the respondents generally felt themselves to be adequately prepared in these fields as far as training and education were concerned.

Criminology

There was a difference of opinion about the importance of criminology between FCNS's and CNS's as it related to their daily work. Most of the CPN's felt that criminology had little bearing on their work whilst 3 of the 5 FCNS's felt that it was an important part of their role.

None of the FCNS's considered themselves to be expert or highly competent in criminology and only 2 rated themselves as being more than competent. Along with the general CNS's, all the FCNS's rated themselves as having little or no formal training in the field. If, as Parry (1991) suggested, a major factor in the speciality of forensic psychiatric nursing is the relationship between crime and mental illness, then the failure of FCNSs to supplement their knowledge of mental illness may warrant further investigation.

Self-awareness

Most people in both sets of CNS's saw self-awareness as being of significant importance to their work, although 2 of the FCN's considered it to be of little or no importance.

It is notable that the idea of self-awareness as a prerequisite for effective psychiatric nursing relationships dates back, rather specifically, to the 1982 syllabus of training for psychiatric nurses. That syllabus was the first to recognise the idea as an important one. It may also be noted that the concept of self-awareness is not a particularly clear one. Nor is there research evidence that we could find that supported the idea that self-awareness really did make a difference to client-nurse relationships.

Research

It was made clear to both groups being interviewed that this section included either the conducting of research or utilising the results of research. While both CNS's and FCN's placed importance on the role of research, none of the respondents considered themselves competent in this area. Of the generic CNS's 2 said that they used research only occasionally or infrequently, this increased to 4 for the FCNS's. This is an interesting finding in the light of the RCN working party (1988) guidelines, stating that the application of relevant research is essential to the role of the CNS. A possible reason for its lack of utilisation could be that the nurses are unable to carry out or evaluate research. Most respondents, in both groups felt that they had little or no formal training in research. These figures support Castledine (1983) who found that few CNS's were able to carry out or evaluate research in a systematic and rigorous way, nor to see the implications of research findings for practice.

This raises questions of how CNS's might develop research skills. First, research training might be included in their basic training. This would have to be of a standard which would allow them to critically evaluate other people's findings and plan and execute their own studies. This would be a considerable undertaking and it must also be questioned as to whether or not such initial training would be feasible.

Second, all CNS's might be offered short courses in research appreciation and in undertaking small research projects. Third, the possibility would seem to exist for CNS's to collaborate with colleges of higher education to enable them to work alongside other researchers who might teach them basic research skills. However, the question arises, here, as to how such joint projects might be funded.

Therapeutic use of security

The FCNS's felt that the therapeutic use of security was more of an important part of their role than did the general CNS's. Moreover, the FCN's had received more formal training in this facet of their role than had the CNS's. However, it might be important that the concept of therapeutic use of security be questioned and challenged. The idea that someone's freedom might be curtailed in order to act therapeutically towards them, seems to be a highly ambiguous one and one that warrants careful definition and discussion. It might be interesting and useful to carry out some observational studies that attempted to identify when such therapeutic use of security was being used.

Social policy

There was a difference in the amount of formal training received in this area, with 2 of the FCN's having at considerable training and 1 having had some. None of the generic CNS's felt they had had formal training in the area. The idea of grounding forensic care in its social context is a vital one. All those who work with offenders do so in a particular social milieu. It would seem important, therefore, that the teaching of social policy in FCPN training courses, becomes a priority. Moreover, it is true that psychiatric nurses who work in the more general field are also meeting clients whose lives are rooted in a social context. It seems, then, that both groups need to address social policy issues even if those issues are different for the two groups of nurses. Social policy issues are also important when nurses make decisions about how to rehabilitate both offenders and psychiatric patients.

Ethics

Both groups of respondents felt that ethics played an important role in their work. There maybe different ethical aspects of care that FCNS's have an interest in, such as control, restraint and seclusion, but this study did not attempt to look into these qualitative differences. It is notable, however, that seclusion and restraint continue to be used throughout the world (Cohen 1988). Some of the ethical issues in this area are discussed in another chapter of this book.

Conclusion

A possible role for the CNS has been proposed by an RCN working party (1988). Bowman (1990) stated that CNS posts have been created largely as a result of medical and public pressure to have skilled nurses supporting medical staff. In such cases nurses are more akin to medical assistants than nurse specialists, as they limit themselves to areas in which doctors are acknowledged to be the holder of the main body of knowledge. If there are to be true forensic nurse specialists their specialist skills and knowledge should be steeped in nursing theory and practice. To attempt to fit psychiatric nursing into the medical speciality of forensic psychiatry would serve to devalue the role of psychiatric nursing and deny its unique contribution to patient care.

The results of this small survey suggest that although some FCNS's place more emphasis on the importance of dangerousness, criminology, and the therapeutic use of security to their work, this is not backed up by a high level of formal training, particularly in criminology and the assessment and management of dangerousness. The lack of education in these areas could be explained by a lack of relevant courses, which in turn could be the result of an insufficient body of nursing knowledge in these subjects, financial resources, awareness of the need for such training and of the underdevelopment of the role.

3 Caring for mothers and babies in secure settings

Sita Devi

A woman who commits a crime and who is mentally well is able to keep her baby with her, albeit in a penal establishment. A women who is mentally ill who has a baby is able to keep her baby if the facility exists locally. However when a female mentally disordered offender is admitted to a medium secure unit no provision is available. With this background in mind it is important to establish the reasons for this. Is that at there is no such need for this facility? Are there no women who are admitted that have babies? Or is that women admitted are considered too dangerous? Would the baby be in danger? Would being admitted to an institution have an adverse effect on the baby? Would it mean that the woman would take longer to recover, because of the pressure of having the baby present? Alternatively, would the women recover more quickly if she was able to have her baby with her?

There has been much published on the importance of the early relationship between mother and baby with the emphasis being that both parties benefit. Bowlby (1969) focused in particular on the attachment between the mother and infant in the first six months of life. He proposed that 'infants were born with a biological propensity to promote proximity and contact with a mother figure'. The word attachment has been defined as an affectionate tie, which endures over a time, binding one person to another. Attachment behaviour ranges is displayed by rooting, grasping and sucking to more advanced levels of

61

a communication system that can maintain contact by crying, gurgling, smiling and calling. Bowlby saw maternal attachment as being the most important type and differing from attachments to other people. Bowlby's early hypothesis was that the 'child's strong attachment to its mother developed during the first six months and was vital for normal, healthy, social development'.

Harlow (1965), in experimental studies of the behaviour of non-human primates, found that baby monkeys spent most of their time clinging to a rug covered teatless dummy only going to the rugless milk giving wire framed dummy when hungry. The baby monkey, not surprisingly grew up, described as ' schizophrenic', 'mentally subnormal' and 'emotionally retarded'. A film of some of his work also demonstrated that male rhesus monkeys when brought up on their own away from other baby monkeys are impotent when adult and a female reared in a similar fashion could not mother its own. Although this research was conducted on non human primates it has been suggested that human would behave in a similar way. Research into bonding may have had benefits for the mother and child in hospital settings. Baker (1961) emphasised that admitting the mother and baby to hospital together minimised the interruption in the mother-baby attachment process by offering treatment within the context of continued family relationships.

This chapter will look firstly at existing literature on mother and baby units and research in this area. A review of the literature shows that many of the worries which are expressed about the safety of the baby have in practise found to be groundless. The benefits however are documented frequently as can be observed through the review of the literature. There is an emphasis that the benefits to both mother and baby together far outweigh the potential costs.

Following a review of the literature, a questionnaire was devised and sent to various Regional Secure Units, prisons and regional mother and baby units to attempt to establish whether the provision of secure mental health facilities in the National Health Service would be further enhanced by adding Mother and Baby facilities to those already present. This involved trying to collate figures about the number of women who would benefit if such a provision existed. The opinions of senior staff on mother and baby units were unanimously of the opinion that secure facilities should include provision for mothers with their babies.

Amongst the senior staff of Regional Secure Units the response was mixed. It is speculated that the reason for this could be that staff on mother and baby units would have a greater awareness of the difficulties in providing care for women who may need some degree of security.

There are presently three mother and baby units within prisons. The security of these vary in each establishment. The three units are at Holloway, Styal and Askham Grange. One of the criteria for admission to the mother and baby unit is that the mother has to be mentally well. If the mother does not fit this criterion the mother is admitted to the psychiatric wing and the baby is taken into care or placed of as the court sees fit. It is unfortunate that at present no figures are available to ascertain how many women are mentally ill, commit a crime and therefore are not considered as suitable for the mother and baby facilities available, within the prison service. It may be that these women at present are being catered for within the National Health Service at existing mother and baby units.

Background

The earliest documentation available of a mother taking her baby with her to hospital was in 1948, when a woman patient from the Cassell Hospital in Surrey asked if she could bring in her toddler, whom she had no one to look after. The medical director T.F.Main agreed to the admission. From this, and subsequent joint admissions, he found two main effects. First, the admission of children helped to maintain and promote the positive elements in the mother/child relationship. Second, mothers were more likely to discuss their anxieties and worries about the mother/child relationship than hide them, if they were allowed to bring the child with them.

By 1955 Main had suggested that to admit a mother solely on her own sometimes colluded with her hostility towards the children and with her wish to be parted from them. Whereas, if children where admitted with their mothers problem resolution was achieved more quickly as the mothers would verbalise their worries and problems to staff instead of avoiding them or hiding away from them. Also in 1955 the Cassell Hospital made it a condition of admission that mothers

63

should bring their babies and children with them whenever possible. The women admitted to the mother/ baby unit tended to have neurotic illness rather than psychotic illness

Baker et al (1957) began to study the problems experienced by young schizophrenic mothers admitted to the Banstead Hospital in Surrey. After a three year study Baker reached the following conclusions. First that to separate a schizophrenic mother from her baby seemed to increase her difficulties and that the case to keep mother and baby together was a good one. Secondly the mother rarely made any attempts to harm the baby, although there was a chance that she may neglect the baby. They also concluded that the mothers' affect towards the baby was normal and that in some circumstances this relationship with the baby was the only normal relationship left. The study also highlighted the difficulty in assessing the mothers' abilities to look after their children. Due to this a recommendation was made that a unit should open for mothers with their babies for treatment, assessment and observation. The unit opened in 1959. One of the first problems encountered by the unit was to establish whether it was possible to treat severely disturbed mothers with their babies. People with severe mental illness were also admitted to this unit. There were no special problems in managing the unit and every patient admitted was discharged home with her baby.

In another study, Grunebaum et al (1961) looked at joint admission of a psychotic mother with baby to a adult psychiatric hospital. They felt the practice of separating mother from baby due to the hospitalisation of the mother-because of mental illness-was based on three considerations (i) the responsibilities of the hospital (ii) therapeutic needs of the mother and (iii) the effects of the psychotic mother on the child. From twelve cases of mother/baby admissions they reached the following conclusions. By allowing the mother to care for her baby the hospital supports the patient in her role as mother. Whereas the practice of separating the mother and baby only reinforce her ideas that she may be harmful to the baby. To give the mother the opportunity to have increasing responsibility for her child, with support and therapeutic interventions tended to make the mother feel less inadequate and guilty. In a therapeutic sense the mother was encouraged and allowed to explore her feelings towards the baby in a safe environment. The mother was able to express positive feelings towards the baby and in this type of setting the staff were able to reinforce those positive feelings.

Grunebaum et al (1963) in a Massachusetts Mental Health Center again highlighted the practice of separating the mother from her baby on admission to a psychiatric unit. They felt that the practice of separating mother from baby rested on four assumptions and involved:

- The mother's inability to deal with her hostility towards the child, who is perceived as a source of demands and threats and who is directly responsible for the mother's acute psychotic reaction.

- That the mother's behaviour, due to her disturbed feelings, fantasies and impaired judgment represents a psychological and physical danger to the child.

- The disturbed behaviour of other patients represents a potential psychological and physical danger to the child.

- The presence of a young child may be disruptive to the ward, the therapeutic management of the ward and therefore harmful to patients.

They looked at the work of Douglas (1956) and raised serious questions concerning the above four assumptions. Douglas (1956) found that mothers with postpartum psychotic reactions were unlikely to relapse if they were given the opportunity to care for their babies in hospital. This report looks at six patients treated successfully in the West Middlesex Hospital and shows that women who are encouraged to assume increasing responsibility for their child in a psychotherapeutic setting, did not relapse.

Grunebaum et al (1963) looked at an individual case of a woman who after having her baby experienced feelings of depersonalisation, ideas of reference and severe anxiety, she was admitted initially on her own. She was hospitalised for six weeks and during this time there was some improvement in her condition and she was discharged. When she returned home she was seen at the Massachusetts Mental Health Centre by a senior staff psychiatrist for follow up care. On her first visit she was found to be seriously depressed and withdrawn. She complained

65

that her mind was weak and that it was full of sand. She was admitted initially on her own and after a month her baby was admitted also. During the mother's and babies stay in hospital Grunebaum and other came to the following conclusions about the original assumptions.

First, it was found that separation from the mother reinforces her fear and resentment of the child and only reinforces her poor self image and renders her feeling inadequate and worthless. To help the mother confront these hostile feeling allows the mother/child relationship to develop and mature.

Second, the assumption was made that the admission of a baby with mother to a psychiatric facility may harm the child. The conclusion reached here was that mothers admitted with their children were better equipped to care for them. If mothers were given responsibility within the care setting, their own feelings of dependency on other people lessened as they were more able to look after their children.

The third assumption, that the disturbed behaviour of existing patients on the ward would affect the child, was not upheld. Patients who wanted to harm the children tended to avoid them. Other patients who attempted to play with the children sometimes frightened them but this may occur in ordinary circumstances when a child meets a stranger. No evidence of harm was found. However, what was observed was the pleasure the children experienced during their contact with patients.

Finally came the question of the management of problems that might occur from having small children on the ward. There were real difficulties involved in helping the mothers care for their children. They also realised that visitors usually had to be over sixteen. However this regulation seemed to disappear and more and more children were observed on the ward. The impression was that the ward seemed more cheerful and home like.

Walde et al (1964) in a pilot study or a joint admission programme established at the Medfield State Hospital, Massachusetts studied nine joint admissions occurring between the Autumn of 1964 to the Spring of 1966. The mothers and their children were admitted to a private room on a closed ward. The children were only admitted after careful social and psychiatric evaluation. Both parents had to agree to the admission of the child and the mother was also obliged to attend regular hospital activities.

The nursing staff were initially apprehensive, they stressed that they had a enough work to do. However, as time passed they became calmer and more motivated. There was concern that the baby may be harmed. Who would take the blame if harm did come to the baby? Despite these anxieties the nursing staff were optimistic about the therapeutic effects of the joint mother/child admission. The physicians expressed similar ideas to that of nursing staff. The primary concern seeming to be who might take responsibility if errors occurred. Given the litigatious nature of the American culture, this focus on responsibility and error is hardly surprising. The majority of patients interviewed were in favour of joint admission. Patients did feel that the mother should be carefully screened and they also felt that a joint mother/child admission would bolster patient morale. There was some concern about the mother actually harming the baby. Some patients felt that the mother should be admitted to another ward with their child and should not be part of the ward community.

Mothers actually taking part in the venture were compliant. They could see no reason for the joint admission yet were happy to go along with it. Only one mother strongly objected to the procedure. In some five cases the relatives strongly objected and the mothers, who in the main were indifferent, sided with the relatives. Most relatives were keen on joint admission apart from the ones documented above. The post admission reactions of nurses were that after the first admission they became increasingly anxious. In the main this anxiety was usually due to the nurses' feeling that the mothers were unable to look after their children adequately. These anxieties soon dissipated.

The reactions of the patients were highly positive on the admission of the first baby. Some patients felt that it made the ward more cheerful. Staff also noted that patients functioned at a higher level for a considerable time after the admission of the first baby. Mothers in the venture expressed positive reactions to the joint admission. Some of the mothers expressed gratitude towards the hospital. Some mothers stressed that the admission enabled them to care for their children more effectively.

Kumar et al (1986) published findings of a survey that they had conducted between 1979-1981. They highlighted the need for planning and co-ordination of services by region. There was a suggestion that day care facilities should also be available as well as a register of national and regional facilities. Crossling et al (1988) in 'Nursing Mentally Ill Mothers With Their Babies', addressed the role of the nurse in the assessment and management of mothers with their babies. Risks such as violence were addressed briefly. Also the particular skills of assessing the mother/baby relationship and the management of specific bonding problems. The Manchester mother and baby opened in 1972 and has since admitted some 600 patients. Mothers and babies are admitted together as it is believed that:

- The mother's prognosis might be improved.

- It is important to maintain the mother and baby relationship and early regular contact is an important part of this process.

- An assessment of the mother's ability to care for the baby is a necessary part of management and may well influence decisions such as time of discharge (Margison, 1982; Margison and Brockington, 1982).

The unit provided beds for nine women with their babies. Each room had the necessary equipment to look after a baby. The unit policy was to allow mothers and babies to spend as much time together as possible. This included babies sleeping in the same room. Babies were admitted as patients in their own right and were examined by a paediatrician on admission. Mothers were assessed in a interview situation to establish the problems that they were facing. A bonding chart was completed twice a day on each patient. For patients that experienced difficulty in expressing themselves verbally they are asked to complete a card sort rating schedule which had been developed on the ward.

One of the problems discussed was the ever present risk of injury to baby especially in the case of the psychotic mother. The risk was assessed by nurses by observing the mother and baby together, the results of the bonding charts for example, handling the baby roughly or being excessively irritable. Psychotic ideas of the mother that could represent harm to the child were also noted.

The bonding chart addressed the following areas: the competence of the mother, the mother's emotional response to the baby, the mother's concern and affection for her baby. The statements that the mother made were noted as were any relevant and special incidents that occurred. There was great emphasis placed on the regular contact of the mother and baby. In psychotic mothers it was found that the mothers' capacity to help with the care of the baby was often an area in which there was least impairment. The bonding chart provided an account of the mothers' behaviour with the baby. The staff found that the lack of mother baby eye contact, poor feeding and absent or mechanical handling of the baby could indicate that there were difficulties in bonding.

The level of intervention from nursing staff was primarily aimed at support, improving practical competence and helping mothers to increase their self-esteem and re-establish confidence. Staff worked alongside the mothers offering support and guidance. The rehabilitation of patients began as soon as it was viable. Mothers were allowed home as soon as it was deemed to be safe enough. These visits home began with a few hours and progressed to weekends. The rehabilitation and preparation of the patients' discharge often involved liaising with community services so that the appropriate support would be available in the community.

Cassell et al (1990) utilised a questionnaire to look at resources available for mothers with their babies. A questionnaire was sent to senior nurses managers in psychiatry in one hundred and twenty hospitals in the south of England and Wales. It was found that mother and baby units existed at 38 hospitals. The conclusions reached were that although there were facilities available for mothers with babies these resources were stretched. Another point highlighted was that if the mother baby unit had five or more beds they were more likely to have specially trained staff and their resources were threatened less. Cassell et al suggested that their findings reinforced the Kumar et al recommendation that there should be a national register for mother and baby units.

Secure facilities

Medium Secure Facilities have been developed over the past fifteen years. In the 1950's there was a shift in mental hospitals from closed institutions to the open door policy. It was found that due to this shift

69

there were a group of patients that could not be catered for in the open hospitals and there were problems finding these individuals appropriate settings. In some cases patients were placed in high security establishments that were not suitable. However they were the only facility available.

In 1961 the Secure Hospital Working Party recommended that regional secure units be provided for these patients. There was little response to this recommendation. The request was repeated in 1974 by the Interim Butler Committee, which looked at the number of abnormal offenders in prisons. The Glancy Committee looked at patients in psychiatric hospitals that needed some level of security. On this occasion these reports met with more support from the authorities. Regional/Medium secure units have been developing since. These units vary in size from a one hundred bedded unit to some that have fifteen beds. The function of the units is the assessment, management and treatment of patients who are considered too difficult or dangerous to be nursed in open psychiatric units. The units are highly staffed on the assumption that this will produce greater therapeutic activity and security with the least personal restrictions possible. The security within these units varies according to the mental state of the individual patient. At present no Regional Secure Unit has a mother and baby facility. Mothers who are admitted through the courts, community or other psychiatric establishments either have their baby taken into care or the baby is looked after by the father.

These are some of the trends in the provision of forensic psychiatric nursing services for mothers and babies. The chapter continues with a description of a small scale study of the views of staff in secure units with regard to such provision.

Sample

A questionnaire was devised and sent to staff in all regional and interim secure units. The questionnaire was also sent to a small sample of staff in prison which were know to have mother and baby units.

Aims of the study

The aim of the study was to sample the views of staff who worked within existing mother and baby units, prisons and secure units. The purpose of this was to establish whether these staff felt that there was a need for secure mother and baby provision within the National Health Service.

Data collection method

The questionnaire was sent to senior nurse managers in all 24 regional secure units, three mother and baby units. A questionnaire was also sent to the psychiatric wings at three prisons. In the prisons the questionnaire was sent to the governor. The survey was conducted by post. The questionnaire was sent to the most senior person within unit.

Data analysis and discussion

A fifty percent response rate was achieved. The response from Regional Secure Units and the prisons was disappointing. The analysis of the questionnaires was carried out by collating all the responses from each item. According to questionnaire returns, the total number of women admitted to Regional Secure Units was 234 in a period of five years where as 956 women were admitted to mother and baby units over the last five years.

Respondents were asked how many women admitted, who had a baby under the age of two, were considered a danger to themselves or others. The data for mother and baby units was separated from the data from the Regional Secure Units. In Regional Secure Units, of the women admitted who had a baby, 83% were considered to be a danger to themselves or others. In mother and baby units, 11% of total admissions were considered a danger to themselves or others. This is understandably a much lower rate to that of Regional Secure Units. However this is what would be expected, as females who would be admitted to a Regional Secure Unit are likely to be more disturbed (by nature of their reason for admission) and therefore much more likely to be considered to be a danger to themselves or others. It would be this aspect that would cause great anxiety to carers when looking at the notion of Mother and Baby Unit within secure units. In other research it has been highlighted that it is very rare for mothers to harm their babies (see, for example, Baker et al 1957, Grunebaum et al 1961).

Respondents were asked on what grounds patients were admitted to mother and baby units. Reasons for admission included puerperal psychosis, pre-existing mental illness for acute phase, assessment for mother and infant bonding, education for mothering skills. Often mothers with neurotic illness had to wait for long periods of time before admission, this may indicate that neurotic mothers may not have the help and support they need.

In Regional Secure Units 84% of women admitted under the Mental Health Act 1983, had a baby under the age of two years In mother and baby units only 20% of women admitted were detained under a section of the Mental Health Act.

Asked whether or not mother and baby units should be developed in secure settings, eight percent said they didn't know. Forty two percent felt that such a service should exist whilst fifty percent felt that such units should not be developed. This pattern of views altered when the data for the RSU's and the mother and baby units was examined independently. In the mother and baby units, for example, all of the respondents felt that a mother and baby unit within a secure setting should exist. While only twenty seven percent of staff in regional secure units felt that such a service should exist. This suggests that once nurses have had experience of this particular client group, they tend to be more positive about the idea of extending the service. On the other hand, those with little or no experience of this facility, seem to doubt the value of it or their own ability to work in such an environment. Also, it seems likely that there is a lack of appropriate facilities for developing such units in secure environments and this may have a bearing on the apparently negative views of the respondents in the forensic settings.

Conclusion

There has been very little research about secure units let alone mother and baby units within secure settings. In this chapter, the author has highlighted some of the issues surrounding the question of whether or not mothers and babies should stay together when the mother is admitted either to a psychiatric unit or a forensic psychiatric facility. As always, more work needs to be done in this important field if the client group are to receive appropriate and humane care. Another question arises from the difference between the two types of facility discussed in this chapter and the resources available for mothers and babies. Stated simply, it is this: whilst psychiatric facilities offer care as one of their main objectives, one of the aims of regional secure units is containment. Thus, it may be assumed that the objectives of the two sorts of units differ. Whilst the former concentrates on helping people to regain health, the later are more concerned with the protection of those outside of the service. Thus, the two units are doing two different jobs and the differences between them should not lightly be glossed over. However, the issue of care versus containment is one that will be returned to in other chapters of this book.

4 Suicide risk in three controlled environments

Neil Kitchiner, Gordon Riach and Anthony Robinson

The question of how secure environments are run is a timely one. Few nurses can be unaware of the particular problems of special units although few nurses are employed in them. This chapter explores some of the special problems of managing people who are suicidal in secure environments. Although the setting is special, the issues discussed are also of relevance to all mental health nurses and to general nurses who care for suicidal patients.

The small study, described in this chapter, was completed in three regional secure units, three prisons and three special hospitals in England in 1990. Staff in areas of each environment were asked to complete a questionnaire designed to ascertain staffs' perception of the observation policy in use when the suicidal person in that environment.

Suicide

There is a considerable literature on suicide which includes that which looks at social trends, the prediction of suicidal intent, studies comparing hospital suicides with other hospitals, but no literature specifically relating to this particular area - regional secure units.

This has meant the material which is referred to in this part of the project is related to suicide and observation but not specifically to

R.S.U's, although much of the literature would appear to link very closely to what is happening today in this area of nursing psychiatric patients, within a controlled environment.

For the purpose of establishing the cause of death, suicide is legally defined as the intentional act of self destruction committed by someone knowing what he is doing and knowing the probable consequences of his actions (Clift vs Schabe 1846). The verdict of suicide has to be supported by evidence: it can never be presumed. Suicide has been reported to exist in every society (Morgan 1984). Attitudes to suicide at a given time and place vary from culture to culture. It can be viewed as a matter of little importance, one of extreme honour or one of mirth. It may be seen as sin or a crime. The ancient Greeks and Romans endorsed suicide in some circumstances (e.g. on behalf of one's country, used as a means of execution in others and in general condoned it except among slaves and soldiers). Suicidal behaviour tends to arouse strong emotional responses in people. The act of suicide is sometimes regarded as `selfmurder' and thus tainted with sin and guilt. The medieval church ferociously condemned suicide and insisted that the soul of a person who had committed suicide was condemned to an eternity in hell.

In the middle ages the corpses of suicides were degraded by being dragged through the streets followed by burial in unconsecrated ground, often at a crossroads with a stake driven through the heart and a stone over the face preventing the spirit from returning to haunt the living (Morgan 1984). As late as 1961, attempted suicide was still a crime in England, where the law made provision for the hanging of the individual, if he she survived. Attitudes have changed since those days and suicidal behaviour is not usually a matter of moral judgement. It has been estimated that every year the equivalent of the population of Edinburgh kills itself (McCulloch and Phillip 1972).

Given that any person may be at risk if stress persistently overwhelms capacity to cope, it is possible to identify factors positively related to self-damaging behaviour. It has been found that on average one third of persons committing suicide have been suffering from a neurosis or psychosis or a severe personality disorder (Stengle 1964).

A common reaction to suicide is to insist that anyone who attempts suicide must be mentally disordered, at least at the time of the act (Kessel and McCulloch 1966). This may divert attention away from situational and social causes of stress. Depressive disorders carry the highest suicidal risk, particularly those with prominent feelings of futility, pessimism, guilt and self reproach. There are individuals who make a rational decision to take their own life. The Roman philosopher, Seneca, commented: 'Just as I shall select my ship when I am about to go on a voyage or my house when I propose to take a residence, so shall I chose my death when I am ready to depart from life'.

Rational suicides seem commonest in persons suffering from chronic, painful and incurable illness. Some 15% of mentally disordered people die by suicide (Guze and Robins 1970). Acute psychiatric illness is the most prominent factor immediately preceding suicide. A large number of suicides, 50%-100% are found to have a psychiatric disorder, many having had periods of psychiatric in-patient treatment (Hagnell and Rorsam 1978). Hospital mortality statistics have shown a recent increase of suicide among in-patients (World Health Organisation 1982) and approximately 1% of all suicides occur within N.H.S. psychiatric hospitals (Mortality Statistics 1985 - H.M.S.O. 1987).

Nowadays we see a shift in attitudes towards prevention (Barraclough et al 1974). Two recent American studies have shown more than 90% of suicides to be mentally ill before their death, and provide a strong case for a medical policy for prevention (Dorpat and Ripely 1977). Barraclough et al (1974) examined the records of a hundred suicides in the south of England. The study identified various clinical aspects of the suicidal patient. It was suggested that suicide is a rare event for those with good mental and physical health. Also it was associated with depressive illnesses, alcoholism, history of past psychiatric treatment, previous attempts at suicide, and evidence of a history of suicide in close relatives. A high proportion of the suicides had given verbal warnings as much as one month before. Suicide therefore is not always a surprise. Barraclough et al suggested some suicides may be preventable, with modern psychiatric treatment, but these methods were not always being effectively deployed.

Hawton (1985) commented that psychiatrists' ability to assess risk of patients killing themselves is probably the most important and demanding of their clinical skills, and one that they often get wrong. I is important to acknowledge that the risk factors for suicide differ according to the group of individuals under consideration.

The risk on acute psychiatric units has been estimated at over 50 times higher than that of the general population, although the risk among all psychiatric hospital patients is considerably lower. Patients with the highest risk are young or middle aged males with affective disorders or schizophrenia, and young females with affective disorders or personality disorders (Pokorny 1964, Copas and Robin, 1982) People are at particular risk if they have a history of previous suicidal behaviour (Fernando and Storm 1984). Risk appears to be increased during the early stages of recovery from illness, where staff vigilance may have lessened (Sletten et al 1972). The position of the hospital has a bearing on suicides. The presence of high buildings or adjacent railway tracks may increase the likelihood of suicidal attempts being made (Langley and Bayatti 1984). The week following admission to hospital and the month immediately following discharge are the periods of greatest risk (Pokorny 1964 and Roy 1982).

A common problem in psychiatric practice is the need to estimate at interview the degree of suicidal risk in a patient: what is the probability that this person will try to kill themselves in the next few hours or days and what factors will alter the risk? (Crammer 1984).

Compared with the outside world, a psychiatric admission ward contains a disproportionate concentration of people judged to be at high risk of suicide. Feeling suicidal is a reason for admission, yet very few patients make the attempt. It seems possible that admission itself reduces the risk of suicide, which may increase again when a patient first goes out on leave or on discharge (Tenroche 1964).

From the literature, it is apparent that suicide is a complex human behaviour that is related to culture, mood, opportunity and to mental health or illness. In the next section, the question of the management of people who want to kill themselves is discussed.

Management of suicidal behaviour

The management of the suicidal patient in most hospital wards whether locked or unlocked is to implement some form of observation of the patient, by the nurses. However patients on special (one to one) or close observation (within sight at all times) may still kill themselves. It has been suggested that special and close observation of the high risk patient is a task for skilled, knowledgable and experienced nursing staff. Rules about the degree of observation required must be simple, clear and agreed by both nursing and medical staff (Salmons, and Whittington, 1989). It would seem important that all nurses who are involved in observing people who are at risk of suicide be trained in such observation. Anecdotal accounts suggest that many student nurses who are asked to observe patients in clinical settings are given few, if any, guidelines about how to do this. Moreover, it has been noted that even general nurses who are seconded to psychiatric hospitals have been asked to observe such patients. It can be imagined that those nurses will have had no training at all in such observation.

Nurses often complain of the stress caused by the presence of the suicidal patient on their units, (Shapiro and Waltzer 1980). The stress they experience in dealing with suicidal patients is often ignored or denied. Dealing with these kind of patients is anxiety provoking for all (Farberow 1967). One assumption when specialing the suicidal patient is that the staff can be and are responsible for the patient's life. Staff members should consciously and conscientiously try to prevent a patient suicide by their presence and actions but at the same time they should realise that despite their best efforts this may not be possible. It is the patient who is responsible for the self destructive act, not the nurse. On the other hand, it might be argued that, given the fact that such patients are deemed to be mentally ill, they are no longer responsible for their actions. It might, thus, be argued that nurses and medical staff must then assume some responsibility for those people's lives. The issue remains, of course, a highly complex ethical issue.

Specialing a patient should be viewed as an opportunity to begin returning control to the patient and use the time to develop the nurse patient relationship. The patient needs to perceive the nurse as being interested in, concerned about, and empathetic to his pain (Blyth M, and Pearlmutter D, 1983). The patient needs concern and help in re-establishing goals so staff should be trustworthy and sympathetic (Pfeffer 1981).

Exploring observation

As already mentioned there is a lack of literature on suicide in regional secure units, although each unit has it's own policy for observing the suicidal patient. Not surprisingly there is a considerable difference from unit to unit. In the three units explored in this small study, the following practices were in operation:

- Chestnut Court RSU operates a three category system whereby a patient is assessed by the medical\nursing staff and assigned to one of the appropriate categories. These include special observation, close observation, or general observation. It is the nurse in charge who is responsible for ensuring that all staff are aware of the degree of observation required for each patient.

- The Oak Court RSU has developed a set of written guidelines for nurses involved in the special continuous supervision and observation of an individual patient. The booklet explains why a special observation might be initiated and gives the nurse clear instructions on what he\she should do. The booklet also gives guidelines for when a patient needs to be transferred to a district general hospital, outlining how the nurses should carry out the continuous observation once there.

- Elm Court RSU operate an individual policy whereby the patient's key worker uses a particular nursing model to assess the patient's level of observation needed.

Aim of the study

The aim of this small study was to examine three nursing environments all of which have facilities for similar types of patients i.e. mentally abnormal offenders.

These environments are all classed as controlled environments because of the way access into and out of them is monitored by specially trained staff. The people who live in these environments are usually detained there either by a section of the Mental Health Act

1983, or at Her Majesty's pleasure. Nine controlled environments were visited to explore how each managed suicidal people. Once all areas were visited and the observation policies collected, staff were asked to complete a questionnaire, aimed at collecting their views about the system they worked with. Finally it was hoped the study would identify areas that should be considered when policy makers draw up guidelines for observation of the suicidal patient.

Collection of data

Once the literature reviews of suicide, observation policies and secure environments had been completed, we were able to draw up a provisional questionnaire. This was then piloted via a group of fourteen charge nurses, nurse tutors, all working within forensic psychiatry. The pilot highlighted some discrepancies with the questionnaire and these were amended before settling for the final draft.

Each establishment was contacted by telephone, to see whether they would be interested in being involved in the study. This initial contact was then followed up with a letter giving a more detailed account of the areas we were interested in looking into, and a date convenient for us to visit. The nine establishments were all visited in one week, and all the information was collected at the time of the visit. The staff who were to complete the questionnaire were selected on the day of the visit by the researchers who attempted to obtain a cross section of different sorts of respondents.

In each of the three areas of each of the three hospitals, we asked one charge nurse and two staff nurses to complete the questionnaire. Respondents were not named after completing the questionnaire but their place of work, and their grade were documented to allow for comparison when analysing the results.

Findings from the regional secure units

All respondents stated that there were facilities, in all three regional secure units, to keep a record of staff's observations of the suicidal patient. There was, however, some variation in the frequency with

80

which suicidal patients were assessed. While most of the respondents reported that such assessment took place on a daily basis, one suggested that it occurred weekly and two others suggested that these assessments occurred at other, unspecified, intervals. Across three units, there was no specified time interval at which the agreed observational policies were to be reviewed. There were also discrepancies regarding the perceived level of observation for suicidal patients. Five respondents suggested that a one-to-one observation regime was applied most often. Three respondents felt that 'close observation' was most often applied, whilst one reported that observation occurred at 15 minute intervals on all suicidal patients. These discrepancies were not linked to particular institutions but were expressed by different people within the same units. This may suggest some confusion about how observation policies are put into operation.

Again, with regard to the staff's knowledge of the observation policies within each of the institutions, there was considerable discrepancy. Four of the respondents stated that they knew the contents of the observation policy whilst the remaining five appeared to be uncertain on this issue. On the question of training for observation of this sort, three staff felt that, in general, staff were adequately trained to cope with the suicidal patient. Another three said that they staff were definitely not trained adequately, whilst the remainder were unsure on this issue.

On the question of who prescribes the level of observation required by any particular, suicidal patient, seven of the respondents said that the nurse was that person. The remaining respondents felt that the doctor fulfilled this role. Two thirds of the respondents felt that their institution were capable of accurately assessing the risk of suicide in their patients but the remaining respondents were of the view that their institutions did not fulfil that role satisfactorily.

Respondents were asked to identify factors that they felt contributed to people attempting suicide within the unit. The list of factors, collated from all three units and in rank order, was as follows:

- Inadequate staffing training.

- Psychiatric illness.

- Staffing levels.

- Inadequate assessment and observational policies.

- Problems with the layout of the unit.

- Level of interaction with others.

- Overcrowding.

- Amount of structure to the patients'/inmates' day.

What such a listing can never offer is the patients' view of what contributes to their wanting to kill themselves. Such a list tends to highlight only organisational and institutional factors, as seen by the staff. If patients were asked to identify factors that contribute to suicide, a quite different list might emerge. In the end, what is of real importance is what the patients' motives are for killing themselves. The listing of organisational factors does not seem to address this central issue. It would be difficult to argue that 'correcting' the above factors would necessarily stop people from feeling suicidal.

These, then, were the findings from the regional secure units. The following two sections describe the pictures that emerged from the prisons and special hospitals.

Findings from the prisons

Three prisons were targeted and for the purposes of this study, these are called Blackstock, Whitestock, Greenstock. It was known that all 3 prisons had experience of suicide, all were of similar (Victorian) design and received prisoners directly from the courts. Whitestock and Blackstock were geographically convenient. Greenstock was though to be a good choice because of the recent amount of media attention it had received concerning suicide. All establishments had hospital services staffed by more than 15 hospital officers and each had at least one full time medical officer. The living accommodation, for inmates, consisted of cellular units without integral sanitation. Inmates dined in their cells

82

and shared that accommodation with at least one other person. The exception to this was the existence of some hospital units where 'single' cells were available.

The respondents were chosen from prison hospital officer grades. Hospital principle officers and governor grades were not asked to directly participate in the study although most were helpful. The researchers were interested specifically in the activities of the 'ground floor' practitioners, those people involved in carrying out day to day interaction with the inmate.

All subjects were assured that any answers given to questions would be treated in strict confidence. Initially, a governor grade from each of the 3 prisons was contacted by telephone and given a brief explanation of the study. Permission was sought and appointments were made to visit the establishments and to talk to respondents. Letters were then sent to each establishment confirming the telephone conversation and re-stating the purpose of the study, including the aims of the research.

The following sections identify the findings from the questionnaire survey. All respondents were aware of the facility to log information concerning the observation of the suicidal patient in the patients' medical notes (as directed in circular instruction 20/1989) and the hospital occurrence book. Respondents also indicated that they not only knew of the procedure for recording suicidal behaviour but also that they used that procedure. The prison differed in the frequency with which they observed potentially suicidal patients. In two of the prison, staff assessed patients on a daily basis. In the third prison, officers claimed to carry out the assessment weekly, although this part of the questionnaire response was not always clear. What did emerge was that a policy had been developed, was used but not always with total consistency in at least one of the prisons. Although circular instruction 20/1989 clearly stated that assessment and observation policies will be reviewed annually, none of the subjects were aware of this mandate. All subjects indicated that they did not know when or who reviewed the policies but all considered that responsibility was with management at higher levels. Subjects from 2 establishments considered that policies were looked at when expedient for 'political' reasons. Neither officer expanded on this view.

It appeared that 15 minute observation was most commonly used in prison as a means of monitoring people who were thought to be actively suicidal. The circular instruction setting out Home Office policy is not specific on this issues and states:

> Inmates thought to be at particular risk of suicide should be placed under special supervision, which may be continuous or intermittent supervision. The purpose of special supervision is to prevent inmates from harming themselves by, observing them or by talking and listening to them in order to alleviate their isolation (Circular Instruction 20/1989 Section E Paragraph 32).

The results show that 7 out of the 9 subjects who participated felt that they had received training in dealing with suicidal patients, however, the precise nature of that training was not specified. However, two thirds of the respondents felt that their training had been inadequate.
The circular instruction governing the implementation of observing and assessing vulnerable patients/inmates in prison is explicit:

> Medical officers should, assess suicide risk on reception and during custody and order prevention measures using Form F1997 (circular instruction 20/1989 section B paragraph 5).

All respondents appeared aware of this and all answered appropriately. Mention should be made however of the hospital officers responsibilities concerning this. Hospital officers are empowered under this instruction to order interim prevention measures when their preliminary assessment suggests an inmate is at risk of suicide, using Form F1996. Two thirds of all respondents felt confident that their own establishment adequately estimated the risk of suicide.

In prioritising factors that respondents felt may highlight inadequacies in assessing and observing those inmates which may have suicidal tendencies it was seen that all felt staff numbers to be most important. When interviewing staff at all 3 prisons it was noted that they were hard working and (certainly at Blackstock and Greenstock) the units understaffed (although this must be acknowledged as a subjective impression). They all complained that due to work demand they were in most cases unable to form relationships with patients/inmates. It was noted that in these three prisons there existed a staffing ratio of three officers to 30 inmates, making a system of individualised care virtually impossible.

Respondents were asked to identify inadequacies in the system of care for the suicidal person. In rank order, these were the factors that were identified:

- Staff numbers.

- Overcrowding.

- Level of interaction with others.

- Physical layout of ward/landing.

- Amount of structure to patients'/inmates' day.

- Psychiatric illness.

- Staff training.

- Inadequate observation policies.

- Inadequate assessment policies.

It is interesting to reflect, on passing, that the accent may be on the prison officers paying more attention to 'keeping people alive' rather than to 'finding out why this person wants to kill himself'. It will be noted, for example, that the first two items in this list are concerned with organisational and staffing issues. Issues such as boredom and psychiatric illness (which might be considered to be more 'psychological') occur only lower down in the list. It is also interesting to note that procedural mechanisms such as observational and assessment policies are not necessarily seen as critical factors. If the prison officers are happy that such procedures are working, then it would seem reasonable that they did not question them as likely inadequacies in the system. However, it will also be noted, that not all of the respondents were completely clear about what those policies were. There is an apparent paradox here. On the one hand, the respondents seemed to be reasonably confident that observation and assessment policies did work. On the other hand, they were unclear as to the nature of those policies. It is also worth comparing the factors identified by the prison officers with those identified by staff in the regional secure units, as described in the early sections of this chapter.

These were the findings from the prison officers; the next section offers findings from the three special hospitals.

Special hospitals

Three special hospitals were then chosen and a similar procedure to that outlined in the previous two sections was carried out to enable the researchers to collect data via the questionnaire (also discussed above. As with the other two elements of the study, three respondents, in three areas of each hospital were invited to take part in the study. Full ethical approval for conducting the study was obtained prior to the distribution of the questionnaire. The three hospitals are referred to as North, South and East hospitals for the purposes of this report.

Findings from the special hospital

In all three hospitals, all respondents were aware that there were facilitates for recording staff observations of the suicidal patient. Also, all respondents noted that observations of suicidal patients were assessed daily. They were less clear about when such policies might be reviewed. Their views ranged from three monthly intervals to annually or infrequently. Many of the respondents did not seem to know when such reviewing took place.

In observing suicidal patients, the respondents were unanimous in their view that suicidal patients were always observed on a one-to-one basis. It was clear from this response that, in the three special hospitals, that meant that a nurse was with the patient at all times.

A large proportion of respondents felt that they had been trained to observe and assess suicidal behaviour. When asked who prescribed the level of observation needed in any given case, in two hospitals, all respondents thought that this was the nurses' responsibility whilst in the third, all thought that this was the responsibility of the medical officer. However, all respondents in all of the hospitals felt that the institution was able to assess the risk of suicide adequately. Overall, there was a feeling that the question of suicide was being addressed adequately in the special hospitals.

When asked to prioritise factors that highlighted inadequacies in observing and assessing suicidal patients, the following, rank ordered list emerged:

- Staff numbers.

- Overcrowding.

- Staff training.

- Special layout of the ward/landing.

- Psychiatric illness.

- Inadequate assessment and level of interaction with others.

- Inadequate observation policies.

- Amount of structure to patients'/inmates' day.

Clearly, staff resource problems were important for both special hospitals and prisons but not so much of an issue in regional secure units.

Discussion

Two points need to be made about these findings. First, the samples used in the three sections of the study were small. Second, the three units cater for different sorts of client groups. To simply compare the staff responses to their client's suicidal feelings, across the board, may produce an odd picture. It must be borne in mind that prison officers are catering for prisoners whilst staff in the other two units are catering for clients or patients who, by definition, are deemed to be suffering from a mental illness. Whilst some of the prisoners may have been designated as mentally ill, this may not necessarily be the case. Also, it can safely be presumed that the overall, institutional aims of prisons, secure units and special hospitals, vary considerably. On the other hand, they are all concerned with the containment of people. This general security element must be as important as the personal security one. That is to say that a prime aim must be to ensure that people remain in the institution. A secondary, but obviously important issue, is the personal safety of those people. This would clearly extend to the prevention of suicide.

Those limitations apart, there are some general points that emerge from this study. First, it would appear that those working in prisons seemed most likely to be clear about procedures for observing and reporting on suicidal people. Second, many of the staff in all three environments claimed that they would appreciate more training in this area and many felt that they had received inadequate training. Also, there were considerable variations with regard to what grade or type of person was asked to carry out the observation and who ordered the observation in the first place.

Factors that were identified as inadequacies in assessing and observing people who were suicidal varied between the different units and these may be noted through reflection on the three lists identified in this chapter. Notably, in the prisons and the special hospitals, staff felt that issues such as overcrowding and staffing levels played a major part here. In the regional secure units, other factors were deemed important. Overall, the study offers brief, but valuable glimpses into the worlds of staff in three different sorts of secure setting. The recommendation is that more research be carried out in this sensitive field.

5   Self-harm in secure environments

Ann Aiyegbusi

To provide purposeful therapeutic experiences for patients who self
harm has long been an aim of professionals working within psychiatry.
Despite this intention it would appear that in practice, professional
action generally falls short of the desired outcome. Forensic Psychiatric
nurses whose role often involves caring for patients who seriously self
harm may find themselves in conflict with their ideals as traditional
approaches to this phenomenon result in little if any observable positive
change in the patients' presentation. It is therefore typical for nurses
who care for patients who self harm to experience feelings of
frustration, exasperation and even helplessness as the activity of nursing
brings little reward in the usual sense. Instead, for the patients there is
an ongoing cycle of emotional distress, self harming behaviours
followed by periods of relative progress which are inevitably followed
by further episodes of emotional distress and self harming behaviours
with no observable means of change may be evident.

The dilemma for nurses may be intensified by difficulty experienced
in relating self harm to either their personal or professional frames of
reference therefore further compounding the problem of successfully
influencing this behaviour by clinical action.

Of the literature relating to self harm, a plethora of descriptions exist
about the range of behaviours and various observable characteristics of
the people who engage in them. Also numerous attempts have been

made to provide insight into the probable function of self harm for patients. For nurses, though, the task of translating this information into a working understanding from which meaningful therapeutic intervention results is a challenging one.

Aims

By scrutiny of the available literature and research in the area of self harm, the study reported here aimed to:-

1. Establish factors which are likely to pre-dispose individuals to engage in self harming behaviours.

2. Offer further insight into the problems experienced by patients for whom self harming behaviour may be just one feature amongst a cluster of psychological and behavioural manifestations of dysfunctional learning experiences.

3. Provide some indicators as to nursing intervention which may enable patients who self-harm to experience needs determined and goal orientated therapy during the period of their lives which is spent within secure psychiatric facilities.

Self-harm

Most studies have observed that more women than men self harm and that typically incidents amongst women tend to involve scratching or cutting the skin causing bleeding, swallowing sharp objects, and inserting foreign bodies into wounds. Incidents amongst men tend to involve striking themselves causing bruising. Incidents of severe genital mutilation have been observed amongst men but this is rarely observed amongst women. In both sexes self harm occurs most frequently during teenage years and early twenties reducing dramatically in frequency after about the age of 30. Most research has been conducted within institutional settings amongst individuals with a wide range of psychiatric diagnoses (Phillips and Allcan 1961, Graff and Mallin 1967,

Rosenthal et al 1972, Simpson 1975, Cookson 1977, Roy 1978, Favazza and Conterio 1988).

When attempting to establish factors which may predispose individuals to engage in self harming behaviour, attention to psychiatric diagnosis is clearly unhelpful. However, whereas self harm occurs amongst patients with a wide range of diagnosis and classifications, the inpatient population appear to be diagnosed mainly as personality disorder and borderline personality disorder (Graff and Mallin 1967, McKerracher, Loughnane and Watson 1968, Gardner and Gardner 1975, Pallis and Birtchnell 1977, Schaefer, Carrol and Abramowitz 1982, Daldin 1988).

By medicalising this phenomenon there is a suggestion that the behaviour is merely the symptom of an illness or condition and not necessarily related to the learning experiences of individuals. When viewed as such, self harm may be interpreted as by Graff and Mallin (1967) who describe the "chronic cutter" whose repeated slashing seems meaningless, unrelated to any maladaptive design, and often unrelieved by environmental changes. Such critical descriptions are not uncommon amongst the literature where the degree to which such patients may prompt negative responses from professionals is often also described. Graff and Mallin (1967) refer to the 'cutter' creating as much hostility as therapy in the hospital setting. Ross and McKay (1979) in their attempts to reduce acts of self harm amongst adolescent girls in a Canadian corrective institution describe, how they blamed the girls for failing to respond to treatment offered, stating that:

in return they gave us crises, demands, complaints, belligerence, insults, belittlement, rejection - and blood.

In a survey of self injury in Holloway prison, Cookson (1977) presents the suggestion that self injury may 'understandably' arouse hostility in the staff who have to deal with it, therefore attention given is of necessity brusque. Favazza and Conterio (1988) describe the 'blood and guts' therapeutic challenge of the chronic self mutilator and here the authors cite feelings of being 'torn apart' and 'emotionally black mailed' as being the experience of therapists who take on this therapeutic challenge. Simpson (1975) suggests that such is the emotional impact of the act of 'cutting' upon medical and nursing staff that the characteristics of the patient presenting the behaviours are often unrecognised.

Undoubtedly the effect of witnessing the results of self harm is often harrowing for professionals, particularly nurses who as a rule initially attend to patients' injuries. This may be coupled with the paucity of information available to provide nurses with a realistic formulation of patients who self harm. It may be understandable that over the decades little has changed with regard to attitudes towards this. In a recent study of deliberate self harming in a British special hospital, Burrow (1992) observes that 'institutional wisdom perceives these 'performances' as the maladaptive, attention seeking malignancy of untreatable psychopaths.'

Rather than relying upon diagnosis to enhance professional understanding of self harm it may be more useful to attempt to establish whether there are significant early learning experiences shared by individuals who engage in these acts and which later serve to shape their personalities and behaviour. Within the literature there is evidence which would support the existence of similarities in the backgrounds of many individuals who self harm. (Simpson 1975, Green 1978, Roy 1978, Carmen Reiter and Mills 1984, Browne and Finkelhor 1986, Shapiro 1987).

Physical abuse

Of the studies which surveyed accounts of experiences during early development, frequent examples of excessive physical punishment were found to be a feature of childhood for a significant number of patients (Roy 1978, Green 1978, Simpson and Porter 1981). Physical abuse of children reportedly occurs in a setting where the child also experiences, scapegoating, alienation, ridicule and humiliation (Green 1978).

Deprivation and neglect

Cookson (1977) found that deprivation of affection was common amongst the inmates of Holloway prison, who self harmed. Maternal deprivation was established by Graff and Mallin (1967). Environmental deprivation and tumultuous families were an experience common in the backgrounds of young male offenders who self harm (Bach-y-Rita 1974). Although Ross and McKay (1979) did not test subjects for evidence of early sensory and social depression they comment about the intriguing possibility of this being a significant factor in explaining self mutilation.

Green (1978) found high levels of self destructive behaviour amongst neglected children. Rosenthal et al (1972) found a 'striking history' of maternal deprivation amongst a population of subjects who self harmed either by cutting or using other means. Interestingly, Mason and Sponholz (1963) observed self-mutilatory behaviour amongst Rhesus monkeys who they raised in either complete or partial isolation - although caution always has to exercised in extrapolating from animal subject to human subjects.

Sexual abuse

In a study of self-mutilation and self-blame in incest victims Shapiro (1987) postulates that self-destructive activity is increased by childhood experiences of violent incestual sexual abuse. It may be surprising then that despite the extensive range of literature about self-harm, hardly has the question of whether subjects have been exposed to sexual abuse been asked. Shapiro (1987) observes that even when the connection between incestuous sexual abuse and self-mutilation is noted, it is buried by papers not directly focused on the correlation. However, some authors have described aspects of their subjects' sexual histories which suggest they may have been victims of sexual abuse. Ross McKay (1979) in their study involving 12 - 16 year old girls observed that many had experienced 'a diet of unrestricted sex during early adolescence'.

Graff and Mallin (1967), when describing the sexual behaviour of their sample of "wrist cutters", note overt incestuous activity amongst some. Bach-Y-Rita (1984) describes the average age of sexual contact as 12 years amongst a group of habitually violent male patients/inmates of a special prison facility who were found to have scars resulting from self-inflicted wounds.

The consequences of childhood abuse

The experience of physical abuse, neglect and/or sexual abuse during childhood clearly results in long-term damage to the victims (Lester 1972, Rosenthal et al 1972, Roy 1978, Green 1978, Simpson & Porter 1981, Carmen, Reiter & Mills 1984, Browne & Finkelhor 1986, Shapiro 1987). This damage, though varying in degree depending upon the nature and extent of the abuse (Green 1978, Browne & Finkelhor 1986) may ultimately leave the victim with chronic behavioural and psychological manifestations consequent to their experience (Carmen, Reiter & Mills 1984, Shapiro 1987). Extraordinary damage to the individuals sense of self culminates in a cluster of clinical characteristics of which the following are reported:

a) Covert experiences

- depression
- chronic anxiety
- impaired self-esteem
- hopelessness
- helplessness
- worthlessness
- guilt
- shame
- experiences of depersonalisation
- feelings of rage and aggression
- episodes of rising tension
- intrusive thoughts
- loneliness
- nightmares
- impulsitivity

b) Social and behavioural observations

- inability to trust others
- sexual adjustment problems
- difficulty forming relationships
- drug, alcohol and substance abuse

- disturbed sleep patterns
- self-harming behaviours
- aggressiveness
- physical expression preferred as opposed to verbal aggression

(Graff & Mallin 1967, Kafka 1969, Lester 1972, Rosenthal *et al* 1972, Bach-Y-Rita 1974, Cookson 1977, Roy 1978, Ross & McKay 1979, Carmen, Reiter & Mills 1984, Shapiro 1987). The characteristics described above are found amongst abused children and also the population of adults who have been observed to engage in self-harming behaviours (Green 1978, Shapiro 1987).

The function of self-harm

The literature supports the view that patients who self harm have generally emerged from childhood with dysfunctional emotional and behavioural coping strategies, ill equipped to survive the demands of adult life. (Green 1978, Carmen, Reiter & Mills 1984, Browne & Finkelhor 1986, Shapiro 1987). Subjectively, the major features of their dysfunction include significantly impaired self-esteem, feelings of depersonalisation, ego function deficits, depressive features and feelings of helplessness and worthlessness. Behaviourally, repeated victimisation, sexual adjustment problems and difficulty forming relationships are likely to reinforce their subjective experiences.

In a study of victims of violence and psychiatric illness, Carmen, Reiter & Mills (1984) found amongst a population of 188 male and female psychiatric in-patients, almost half had histories including sexual and/or physical abuse. In this study it was observed that abused patients dealt with emotions such as anger differently from non-abused patients, females most frequently internalised anger and aggression and engaged in self-harming behaviour. These patients were described as most depressed, withdrawn and felt worthless, helpless and undeserving of treatment. The females were described as victims during childhood and this continued throughout their adult lives within the relationships they had.

In terms of the function self-harming behaviours serves for the patients who engage in it, there is overwhelmingly consistent reporting of a frequent sequence of experiences common to those who self-harm and during which self-harming occurs. Typically these are feelings of numbness or depersonalisation which may continue until the patient self-harms. Self-harming reportedly brings about the experience of re-integration, then a return to reality and a reduction in tension occurs coupled with an increased sense of self. (Kafka 1969, Lester 1972, Rosenthal *et al* 1972, Bach-Y-Rita 1974, Gardner & Gardner 1975, Simpson 1975, Cookson 1977, Simpson & Parker 1981, Carmen, Reiter & Mills 1984, Brown & Finkelhor 1986, Farazza & Conterio 1988, Burrow 1992). Because of the efficacy of self-harm in its ability to reduce feelings of tension for the individual in the absence of alternative coping strategies, the acts serve as positive reinforcement here. The result being that behavioural change is difficult to achieve.

There is some evidence which supports the view that there is a secondary gain for patients who self harm, especially when they are detained in conditions where little opportunity exists for exerting control over environmental events. Penal establishments, special hospitals and secure psychiatric facilities as well as general psychiatric hospitals would usually be included (Bach-Y-Rita 1974, Cookson 1977, Ross & McKay 1979, Franklin 1988). Within these settings, antecedent events of interpersonal conflict, thwarting and disappointment are reported. Also, increased self-harming behaviours have been observed during periods of isolation, boredom and inactivity. Ross & McKay (1979) cite a statement from one of the female adolescent self mutilators in their study who described how by "carving" the girls controlled the 'Grandview emergency machine' by setting in motion a chain of events.

The supervisors called the head supervisors, the head supervisor called the duty administrator, the administrator came running and summoned a retinue of professionals - the nurse, the doctor (if you cut deeply enough), the ambulances (if you really do it right), the male staff (if you are obstreperous about it or keep cutting instruments in view), and even the psychiatrist (if you threaten to keep doing it) (Ross and McKay 1979).

Nursing intervention

As has previously been suggested, the often extreme nature of self-harming acts and the consequent experience of carers as a result of witnessing episodes, may limit the perception of the patient's clinical presentation to the most pronounced behavioural excess i.e. self-harm. Clearly, nursing interventions which focus directly upon the self-harming behaviours in isolation of other areas of need on the patient's part are unlikely to be effective in the long term. Reactive restrictive practices such as physical restraint, seclusion, restraint garments and restriction of movement appear to have little value in terms of reducing the extent to which self-harming behaviours occur in individual cases or amongst groups (McKerracher, Loughane & Watson 1968, Simpson 1975, Cookson 1977, Ross & McKay 1979, Aldridge 1988, Burrow 1992).

In the study of deliberate self-harming behaviour of patients in a British special hospital, Burrow (1992) most poignantly highlights the fact that at the time of the study, the excessive degree to which self harm was evident at that hospital:

Is contingent upon a regime which fails to engage a sufficient, negotiated participation of it's client group [and] a reduced capacity for personal adaptive strategies, derivational origins and a limited repertoire of institutional responses to their dilemma all conspire to disadvantage seriously women in such an environment (Burrow 1992).

In the Ross & McKay (1979) study of the 'Grandview carvers' after reviewing a number of possible therapeutic interventions and implementing several ingenious strategies of the authors' own design, self-harm significantly declined amongst the young female subjects when the researchers had unwittingly involved the subjects in prosocial means of controlling their social environments.

Later, when identified as such, the researchers strategically set about 'co-opting' subjects to co-ordinate their peers in a manner which promoted prosocial behaviours to exert control over their lives within the institution. During the period of time that this intervention was operational, all self-harm at Grandview remained diminished.

Aldridge (1988) viewed self-harming behaviour as a systemic phenomenon in the context of a psychiatric hospital ward and eliminated it from that clinical area by involving both staff and patients in a strategy for resolution. This involved scrutiny of the behaviour of all parties in order to see how the system was organised. This was followed by the facilitation of negotiation and consultation amongst all concerned as means of resolving the common problem and formulating a common goal. Possible solutions were proposed rather then imposed and agreed policy was consistent and based on concrete rather than previously abstract actions. Patients were each assigned a named principal therapist who would then co-ordinate all therapeutic strategy for that patient and all others would then refer to this individual. Because of previously prevailing anxiety related to the possibility of one of the women killing herself, death was openly discussed and patients encouraged to express their desires as to what should happen to their affairs following death. In the event of self-harming behaviours occurring, no attempts were made to stop patients from engaging in them and crises were avoided. In an attempt to legitimise the women as people in their own right, their individual biographies were reframed in such a way as to provide staff with a greater understanding of the patients' predicaments and so the past was used to explain the present. After eighteen months, no self-harm occurred on that ward.

It seems then that the elements of nursing actions most likely to provide meaningful therapeutic experience for patients who self-harm involve empowerment of patients to effect environmental change and circumstance. Also, for nurses to implement clear and consistent interventions which target identified needs as expressed by patients. In so doing, validation of previous experience which has culminated in such extreme acts in order to resolve conflicts should occur. It would then follow that interventions which ultimately enable patients to express emotion in a less damaging manner, training in anger and/or anxiety management, interventions to raise self-esteem and strengthen ego structures are likely to be indicated for most. By focusing upon those areas of need which appear to be common to most patients who self-harm, the actual instances of this behaviour are likely to reduce

(Ross McKay 1979, Carmen, Reiter and Mills 1984, Shapiro 1987, Aldridge 1988, Feldman 1988, Burrow 1992).

Discussion

Although self-harm is generally just one feature amongst a cluster of other clinical symptoms experienced by patients who engage in the behaviour, it is often perceived by carers as somehow overriding others. Undoubtedly this is as a consequence of the extreme and often dramatic responses such behaviours elicit. Such responses may take the form of interpersonal reactions from individuals and also the extent of environmental change which may occur, often when the patient has little else available with which to prompt such activity.

This chapter aims to emphasise the likely cause and function of self-harm particularly within secure or controlled environments. In doing so, it is necessary to point out that there still remain areas in which nursing practice generally appears to fall short of meeting the needs of patients who deliberately self-harm in such environments. It seems that if this situation is to improve, considerable research is indicated. Recommendations as to the nature of such would be directed towards attempting to establish a package of care which involves a systematic approach to resolving the deficits which appear to be common to this particular patient group. Such a package may require a valid assessment tool from which Forensic Psychiatric nurses could determine specific and measurable areas of need.

In order to implement actual nursing interventions which enable patients to progress, both further research and training are indicated. Research, would aim to specify those interventions which are most useful. Training is required to enable the skills necessary to employ interventions which are readily available for patients as and when they are needed. This is likely to be constantly and consistently. Whilst other professional disciplines and specialist nurses may be equipped with the necessary expertise, it is probable that this may be on a sessional basis. As nurses generally provide twenty four hour care, it may be appropriate for such patients to receive twenty four hour clinical expertise.

A further area where research appears to be indicated it that of whether patients who self-harm are likely to be best treated as individuals amongst patients experiencing a variety of mental health problems. Alternatively, whether specialist facilities are indicated whereby groups of individuals sharing similar problems should be treated together as is currently the practice with drug and alcohol abusers. If so, the question should be posed as to whether such facilities would specialise in the care and treatment of people who self-harm, or rather, in the care and treatment of victims of abuse as this may well be the root cause, fundamental to the presenting problems and possibly a more accurate indicator as to care needed.

6 Nursing management of fire risk in controlled environments

Andrew McGleish

Nurses are often in the position of making decisions about patient care which may involve a risk of harm to the patient or to others. Carson (1988) suggests that 'risk-taking can be the essence of professional responsibility.' To avoid risk-taking may avoid the possibility of harm occurring but will also prevent any benefits from being felt. However to take appropriate risks we have to have the ability to recognise and weigh up the competing factors.

Nurses in Regional and Interim Secure Units work with mentally disordered offenders and patients who have proved to be too difficult to care for in other psychiatric hospitals, but do not need the maximum security of a Special Hospital. While many of the patients will have been referred with an index offence of an assaultative nature, a minority will have been referred because of deliberate fire setting (see Treasaden 1985)

With such a client group it could be expected that nurses in this field would be expert at judging the risks. Yet any visitor to these units will quickly pick up upon the many and varying practises which abound in the name of security or safety. This variety of practises possibly reflects the relative youth of this service and the scanty information published which could be of use in making decisions of policy. Menzies (1959) suggested that the use of ritualistic nursing tasks operates as a socially structured defence against the anxiety provoked in the nursing situation.

One may not require a psychoanalytical approach to speculate on the strength of anxiety possible when working in secure units.

Some units place importance on banning items which are perceived of as constituting a serious danger. Part of their management of risk thus involves blanket policies which cover all patients, staff and visitors. This means that the patients, whose life is already controlled and limited by virtue of being detained, may find that they are denied access to everyday items, not because of any problem that the individual may have but because of a blanket policy.

The dilemma that nurses face is that of maintaining the safety of patients, staff and the public, whilst caring for the patients in the least restrictive manner possible. The essence of this dilemma is that in order to evaluate the progress or needs of patients, they have to be put in the position of having enough control over events to behave in the way that they would choose. This implies, to this author, that there has to be the possibility of repeating, in some way, the behaviour that precipitated admission in the first place.

The potential danger that fire represents is one that most nurses will be aware of and have respect for. It is a force which appears uncontrollable and unpredictable and is perhaps removed from the daily concerns of most. Yet nurses in many settings may be involved in assessing patients' ability to safely manage fire hazards.

This project examined a problem which highlights the dilemma faced by nurses in Regional Secure Units. Blanket policies which ban matches and lighters for patients within the unit are often seen as a commonsense precaution against what is perceived as an increased risk of fire. Does this prove to be sufficiently effective that the use of individualised control could be seen as negligent?

The question of how nurses in Regional Secure Units make decisions about their own practise and as part of Multi-Disciplinary teams is something which requires a lot of research. Greater knowledge about the probability of dangerous behaviour occurring would be important, not just in terms of providing environments which are appropriately therapeutic and controlling but in the future management of and provision for this client group.

Background literature

Stollard (1983) identifies five fire safety tactics; 'Ignition Prevention', 'Fire Control', 'Egress', 'Refuge' and 'Rescue'. The tactic which this project concentrated on was that of Ignition Prevention since this appears to be the area where the problem is seen to lie in the Regional Secure Units. Nurses searching the literature will find little written by other nurses on the problem. Perry (1991) wrote a care study of his work with a patient on a regional Secure Unit for Mentally Handicapped Offenders. He described the, apparently successful, use of Behaviour Modification techniques with a young woman using the model proposed by Jackson, Glass & Hope (1987) which will be discussed later.

Two articles about Regional Secure Units, both written by nurses, give differing perspectives on how firesetting is viewed. Rix and Seymour (1988) describe a survey of violent incidents in which fire setting was classified, for the purpose of their report, as a minor violent incident, of the same level as self injury or 'violence which is threatened, but not inflicted'. However, Quinn (1979) mentioned that a patient was 'accepted without question in a Special Hospital after he set a fire in the ward.' (p240) Neither of these articles were written about fire risk problems but do throw some light on practise on Secure Units.

Most of the published output by nurses tends to discuss the need to be well prepared for the event of fire. Wyatt (1985) discusses the problems caused by not knowing the 'Fire Drill' during a real fire. Rosenthal and Rosenthal (1988) discuss the far-reaching effects of a hospital fire, paying a lot of attention to the economic costs. Frickman (1973), a psychiatrist, makes the point that patients should have their doors 'tagged' if they are in seclusion.

Tousley (1985), again discussing plans for responding to fire, asserts that:

> provided that nursing approaches to them are the same, behaviour patterns of psychiatric patients during a fire are consistent with past behaviours. If the staff remain calm, so will the patients.

This article, like the others before it makes no attempt to use anything other than anecdotal evidence to support the author's assertions. Mieszala (1982) provides the only other article by a nurse which addresses the problem of Arson. This appears to be directed at nurses working in the 'Burns care' specialism. She refers to differing classifications of motive, concentrating on 'Arson for profit' and 'Pyromania'. Intervention with Juvenile fire setters receives special attention, Mieszala stating that the key factor in this is 'early identification of the firesetting behaviour as an expression of need.' Whilst all but writing off the adult 'Pyromaniac' as untreatable, ('Arrest and punishment (or treatment) often meet the pyromaniac's need for attention'), she makes the point of pleading for a change in attitude in those who deal with children. Three questions are proposed which are claimed to have particular relevance to answering the larger question of 'Why did you set the fire?':

- What does the firesetting do for the person, whether child or adult?

- What are the person's general needs (as seen through lifestyle, environment, social development and so forth?

- What are some other less dangerous ways of meeting the persons needs? (Mieszala 1982).

Mieszala argues that an approach based around these factors is most successful with children in the 2-6 age group. The diagnosis of Pyromania and resulting pessimism about treatment possibilities for adults is dealt with later on in this review.   Gaston (1982) described a programme which was aimed at tackling the 'smoking incompetency' of the patients on a long-term ward. The staff completely controlled the patients access to their cigarettes and matches while they were on the ward and provided an area in which smoke breaks could be taken. This not only resulted in a reduction in the amount of fire damage but an increase in the therapeutic interaction between the patients, staff and professionals.

Whilst the 'incompetent smoking behaviour' had been identified as the problem which required intervention, the programme appeared to be as much about improving the relationships between the untrained ward staff, patients and the professionals who had responsibility for the ward. One problem which Gaston identified was the reluctance of the untrained staff to use anything other than cigarettes as interventions in disturbed or agitated behaviour. Providing the skills necessary to make more therapeutic interventions and building trust between the staff and professionals allowed more individualised approaches to care under the guise of a 'blanket' policy.

The report of the committee investigating the fatal fire at Warlingham Park Hospital (Warlingham Park 1982) suggested that patients should be searched for smoking materials at night and the same stored in a secure area. This was one of 20 recommendations made by the committee. Barker et al (1991) survey fire incidents in two linked psychiatric hospitals and suggested that fire incidents have many similarities to violent incidents. Their relative infrequency points to thew need for long term prospective research.

The remainder of the literature refers to the Arsonist or deliberate fire-setter, this author will use the term fire-setter as a generic term, unless quoting others, because of the specific legal meanings of the terms 'Arson' and 'Arsonist'.

Fire-setting

Soothill (1990) argues the difficulty of detection for the crime of Arson and points out that much of the research on Arson will involve a biased sample of offenders, ie, those who have been caught. He reminds the reader that

> the major danger is to suggest that arson as a general problem lies in the province of the psychiatrist...for psychiatrists tend to restrict our understanding of what is essentially a social problem.

Research by Kafry (1980) suggests that interest in fire was almost universal in a sample of 99 'normal' young boys and that fire play was carried out by 45% of them. This would suggest that setting fires was not in itself abnormal at that age group. The problem of 'match play' was not isolated but was found to be related to other problems, these boys were noted to have come from the more deprived families in the sample. Vreeland & Levin (1980) offer a useful overview of psychological aspects of firesetting, from arson for profit through solitary firesetters to group firesetters. They note that arson for profit is mostly ignored in the psychiatric literature because of it's apparently rational motivation. It is suggested that the psychological factors which encourage, for example a business person to turn to fire to solve economic problems is an area that needs more research. After discussing the various other groups and theories of motivation for firesetting, they conclude with an argument for further research into the hypothesis that firesetters are socially ineffective and avoid activities which will involve confronting another person. The lack of data about treatment procedures was also noted as presenting opportunities for further research.

Prins et al (1985) proposed an eleven point classification scheme for Arson which appears to include childhood, amongst other things, as a motive for fire raising. What they do point out is the complexity of motives involved in the crime. Geller & Bertsch (1985) searched the records of all 'non-geriatric' patients in an American state hospital and found that 26% of them had been involved in some form of fire setting behaviour. Of those half had only engaged in this behaviour once. This article is useful in that it does not depend upon previously identified firesetters but rather examines the whole psychiatric population of one hospital. They note that those who had exhibited firesetting behaviour were also more likely to have had more or longer admissions to the state hospital and to engage in non-lethal self-injurious behaviour. They raise the concept of:

> Firesetting behaviours as forms of communication directed to known others and as examples of destructive operant behaviour (Geller & Bertsch).

However they point out that 'the nature of fire renders it dangerous to, others and hence makes the psychiatric patient/firesetter feared'. They conclude by describing firesetting as a:

> ...dangerous behaviour of the worst kind for a practising clinician; unpredictable, infrequent and highly lethal.

Epidemics of fire setting in mental health units have been described in two separate papers. Boling & Brotman (1975) describe a situation where 13 fires were set by four patients over a short period. None of these patients had a history of fire setting and the authors link the epidemic to institutional conflict which prevented 'key personnel' from making firm administrative stands. They go as far as saying that the 'choice of fire setting as a mode of expression appears to resonate with the feelings of the staff in regard to the state of the institution.'

Rosenstock et al (1980) presented a similar picture, from a systems perspective, of problems with the handling of crises on a unit engendering an epidemic of fire setting. Whilst the patients involved had several features indicated in the personalities or personal histories of known fire setters, none had any previous history of fire setting. Their recommendations include advice on the management of individual patients involved as well as advice on the social factors and pressures within the unit as a whole. Before moving on to look at that literature which deals mainly with the firesetting individual it is worth considering the use of fire in self harm attempts. A report of nurses being sued in America (Regan Report 1985) hinges around the fact that nursing staff did nothing to control a patient's access to lighters after she had made repeated attempts to set fire to herself. Soni Raliegh et al (1990) showed that almost 30% of the suicides of Indian women in England and Wales were by burning. This is possibly related to the practise of 'suttee' by Hindu women in parts of India.

Research carried out amongst in-patients at the Maudsley Hospital, London by (Jacobson et al. 1985) suggests, amongst other things, that "the general method of self-harm used may be less important than the features in common in the chronically suicidally ill.' Over a nine year period 10 patients had used fire in one self harm act each. This is out of 254 patients who had committed such acts and of a total of 592 acts. The authors provide some useful advice for those caring for such a vulnerable population but do recognise the limitations of their study.

Dooley (1990) found that out of 346 suicides and consciously inflicted deaths in prisons over a fifteen year period, 10 had been due to fire. The difference between the two classifications is that of intent to die, and it was found that proportionately more of the consciously inflicted death group died using fire. Power & Spencer (1987) found 8% of cases of 'parasuicide' in a Scottish Young Offenders institution to be based on firesetting of cell items. Holley & Arboleda-Florez (1988) argue that self-destructive behaviour in prison can only be explained by taking into account the social structure of the prison and by viewing the act as a means of gaining some control over the prisoner's own life.Those prisoners who are unable to abide by the rules and regulations of prison life will be more at risk. Finally the suggest that punitive responses to these inmates may increase the likelihood of more dramatic and serious self-destructive behaviour ensuing.

All of the above would suggest that fire may be used in self harm attempts by a minority of those who may make this kind of act. The samples are all too small to compare, eg, the difference between prisoners and hospital patients. The choice of fire is however noted to be worrying since it is unstable and unpredictable.

Pyromania?

Crossley & Guzman (no date) surveyed psychiatrists in the Canadian province of New Brunswick, and found that out of all the arson related cases presented to them only 2.9% were diagnosed as Pyromaniac. The criteria used for this diagnosis was that of the Diagnostic and Statistical Manual of Mental Disorders, third edition (1980)(DSM III) as follows:

- recurrent urge to ignore impulses to set fires;

- increasing sense of tension before setting the fire;

- an experience of either intense pleasure, gratification or release at the time of committing the act;

- lack of motivation such as monetary gain or socio-political ideology for setting fires;

- no evidence that firesetting was due to organic mental disorder, schizophrenia, anti-social personality disorder or conduct disorder (DSM III).

Harris & Rice (1984) devote considerable space to the psychoanalytical approaches to the problem and find that in the early works much emphasis was placed on the same few case studies, rather than on any large scale research, to formulate fire-setting as a sexually motivated problem. This resulted in the impression being given that a lot was known about it. They summarize the previous literature as follows:

Cases presented are those which fit the explanatory approach of the authors; treatment is seldom discussed; motives provided by the arsonist are not seen as credible; and sexual motives are almost always asserted to be involved, at least under the surface. Firesetters are said to be dangerous individuals who should be institutionalized for very long periods.

This strong refutation of a long tradition of psychiatric and psychological work with firesetters requires a strong alternative explanation to follow it. These authors describe a study they carried out comparing arsonists with other offender patients at a maximum security hospital. The results of this survey showed that arsonists are less assertive than other offender patients. They described themselves as having less control over their lives and were rated as less assertive on behavioural tests. These assertion deficits were shown to be 'obvious and substantial' and not an artifact of the tests. They conclude by stating that:

Psychodynamic accounts of firesetting behaviour may explain, at some level, the behaviour of interest, but they do not provide an understanding of the phenomenon that can be used to design treatment.

Other writers have addressed the theme of firesetters as lacking in social skills. Hurley & Monahan (1969), in a study of prisoners at Grendon Underwood prison, found that in comparison with the 'normal' population arsonists exhibited gross social dysfunctioning. When compared with other offenders at Grendon who showed a similar picture in social ability, the arsonists had a different offence pattern with more property damage offences and fewer of 'false pretence'. A high frequency of disturbed family background, poor school and work records, sociosexual problems, alcoholism and attempted suicide was noted.

In contrast with part of the above, Hill et al (1982) found that arsonists in their study were a mixture of property and violent offenders, with the most frequently recognised motive being revenge with underlying anger. The most frequent victims were institutions rather than individuals and most of the arsonists were unable to verbalize their reason for setting the fires.

Jackson, Hope & Glass (1987) compared arsonists with other violent offenders and a control group at the then Moss Side Hospital. Again, although many similarities were found between the arsonists and violent offenders, the arsonists group rated themselves as significantly less assertive than did the other groups. The arsonists also had more difficulty in gauging the seriousness of different offences against property or people.

The role that alcohol plays in the lead up to an act of fire setting is pointed out by Yesavage et al (1983) and Koson and Dvoskin (1982). The high incidence of family, personal and situational stress was noted in both papers. In Koson & Dvoskin this was particularly so of the recidivists or repeated offenders. They end their paper by asserting that firesetters should be recognised as '...dangerous...with a need for control, limit setting and scrupulous long-term supervision and follow up in the community.'

A high recidivism rate of 35% by fire setters studied in prisons and psychiatric hospitals in South West Ireland by O'Sullivan & Kelleher (1987) contrasts with the results found by Sapsford et al (1978).They found a rate of only 5 or 6% of reconvictions for Arson, however this figure was seen to increase to 20% of those considered to be more serious offenders.

O'Sullivan & Kelleher (1987) also noted a high rate of self harm and suicide amongst the group that they studied.

Jackson, Glass & Hope (1987) attempt to describe a model of recidivist arson based on their own clinical experience and the literature on the problem. This model uses a framework of 'Functional Analysis' which is intended to examine a problem behaviour and establish the relationships between the behaviour and the different variables linked to it. This will be familiar to psychiatric nurses in the shape of the 'ABC' approach (Antecedents-Behaviour-Consequences). The formulation presented is that:

110

Arson is viewed as an attempt to exert a change in the arsonist's life conditions where alternative behaviours have proved, or are perceived to be, ineffective (Jackson, Glass & Hope 1987).

Among the Antecedents identified are the three settings of:

- personal and environmental (psychosocial) disadvantage;

- dissatisfaction with self and/or life;

- actual or perceived ineffective social interaction.

Previous experience of fire (possibly involving significant emotional events or obvious social effects) and inhibition of alternative behaviour may direct the person to the use of fire. The triggering conditions involved may include, opportunity and/or the absence of an identifiable 'person target', and a situation which is emotionally significant and induces conflict between the need to change and the inability (perceived or actual) to actually change it. While admitting the speculative nature of several components of their analysis they propose that future research be done to validate and refine the model. Where this model appears to be useful is that it takes into account the situation that the patient finds him or herself. This can then indicate possible avenues to explore in intervention with the patient.

Treatment

In one of the few modern articles to relate firesetting to sexuality, Bourget & Bradford (1987) describe the treatment of two male patients for whom fire had become a fetish. Pharmaceutical and behavioural treatments were used with some success , although one patient did not cooperate when discharged to the community. Other examples of treatment include the work done by Rice & Chaplin (1979) based on the use of social skills training to counter the identified assertive deficits. This had not been fully evaluated but did show that one year after the treatment eight of the patients involved had not been caught or suspected of Arson.

The Rehabilitation Centre at Ashworth Hospital (South) (Ashworth 1990) runs a course of Arson treatment groups, based on the work of Jackson, Glass & Hope(1987), although this has yet to be evaluated.

Summary

The literature available provides little to guide nurses planning the fire safety tactics to adopt in the setting of a Regional Secure Unit. Next to nothing has been written which actually addresses the concerns of the day to day care and treatment of 'forensic' patients nor of those who are regarded as firesetters. The literature on firesetting is divided amongst those who regard firesetters with the gravest of doubts for their future prognosis because of some intra-psychic deviance while others take a more optimistic view. Little is available which will allow predictions to be made about future behaviour or assessment of current needs. The work by Jackson, Glass & Hope (1987) appears to be the most useful to nurses, offering a model for individual assessment and care planning. This model has the benefit of being open to use by people who work within different theoretical frameworks, eg behaviourism or psychodynamics.

However it has to be recognised that most of the work available is based on small scale studies of disparate groups and themes picked up from the work of others in similar positions. What is clear however, is that firesetting should not be viewed solely as a behaviour exhibited by individuals who 'get a kick out' of fires but rather that a myriad of factors may be involved. Of importance may be the social environment created on the unit. Issues of empowerment and control are identified in several articles related to both self harm and fire setting. A link between self harm and firesetting has been noted in several articles.

That people have not been known to set fires previously is not a guarantee that this may not become a problem although this may only be relevant for a few individuals. Again previous firesetting may not necessarily be a good indicator for the future. This leaves us in the position of being unable to say with any scientific certainty whether our care and treatment will be successful in even the short term. Nurses in secure units have an opportunity to actually create a body of knowledge for clinical practise which could be innovative amongst all disciplines.

Aims of the study

The aim of the small study described here was to survey the Regional Secure Units in England to examine patterns of fires and also compare fire rates between those units which pursue blanket bans on matches and lighters, and those which pursue more individualised policies.

Methodology

The project was carried out with questionnaires being sent to the Senior nurses of twenty Regional and Interim Secure Units in England. The questionnaire was devised in two parts. The first was intended to provide raw data about policies, fires, size, total number of admissions, length of time open, and number of patients admitted with reason for referral as arson or fire-setting. In particular the first question was phrased to examine whether the unit pursued a blanket policy of banning patients from carrying matches and lighters within the secure area of the unit. Questions were also included to detect those units which had made a change in their policy which would affect the results.

The second part was intended to provide information about the nature of the fires on Secure units, with the intention being to compare those results against studies of fire in other hospitals. The classifications were adapted from a fire classification system proposed by Stollard (1983, 1984, 1984/85). This classification system was used in his study of hospital fire reports. Changes were made in order to provide data in a manner which could throw light on the aim of the study and on the problem in general.

The main change was in the classification of 'Sources of Ignition'. Stollard (1983) included 'Malicious' as a source of ignition and grouped together matches, lighters and other smokers materials. This author divided matches, lighters and other smokers materials into discrete items. A different set of categories were created to examine the nature or cause of the fire (as opposed to source of ignition). This was introduced in the hope that more information could be provided which could be of particular interest to nurses. For example, 'self-harm' would have been included by Stollard under malicious or deliberately started fires. However the frequency of the deliberate use of fire in self harm

113

attempts may have implications for nursing practise.   Respondents were asked to provide information from the time that their unit opened to the present. This approach was felt to be more useful since, as the sample was by its nature small already, further limitation by specifying for example two years would have provided very few incidents of fire.

The questionnaire was then given to various course members to check if the questions were understandable and valid in their experience.

Findings

Replies were received from fifteen of the twenty units which were sent the questionnaire, a response rate of seventy five percent. Five units indicated that they had a blanket policy of banning all patients from carrying matches and lighters within the secure area of the unit. Ten indicated that they did not use such a policy. Some respondents commented on the reason for, or particular facets of, their non-blanket policy. Of the total replies, two units responded that they had changed their policy; one to a blanket ban after several malicious fires, the other from a blanket banning policy to one in which some patients would be allowed to carry matches or lighters. The results from these two units are not used for the purposes of comparing data about the effectiveness of a blanket policy.

Three of the units were unable to provide figures about patients admitted with an index offence of arson or with a reason for referral given as fire setting. Of those units which had the information, and had no policy change, the overall rate was 7.4%. The figures for units with the ban policy and those without are 6.1% and 8.7% respectively.

Three units had no fires, the rest having between one and seventeen fires. Analysis of the baseline data from each unit, in terms of policy, size, age, admissions and fires, showed only one obvious measure which could be used to compare the effect of the 'ban' policy. This would be the rate of fires per admission. This figure was achieved by dividing the sum of fires by the sum of admissions. The results from this showed that the rate of fires per admission for those units with the ban policy was 26 fires over 1093 admissions. The rate of fires per admission for the units without the ban policy was 32 fires for 1384 admissions. This actually shows a slightly higher rate of fires per admission for those units which ban patients from carrying lighters and matches. If taken over 100 admissions the rate is virtually the same.

As was shown earlier those units which did not operate a blanket policy actually recorded a slightly higher overall rate of patients with reason for admission as arson or fire-setting. Since not all units provided the necessary information and the sample is so small, this cannot be taken as definitive but does suggest that on the basis of the patient groups the comparison is of like with like. A more in depth analysis of the patient populations would be necessary to establish whether different units did have a trend of admitting patients who posed a higher degree of risk.

One criticism of these figures would be that of those units which do not operate a blanket ban, some of the larger units may have different policies for different wards. Thus patients in, for example, an admission ward would not be allowed to carry matches or lighters, but would be allowed to on other wards. This would mean that rather than operating individual assessment and implementation of nursing care, the units would be operating only a more selective blanket policy.

This criticism could be tackled by examining the figures from the small units which consist of only one ward. These units would then depend totally on individualised assessment and implementation. The results from this show a slight change in the results, with the figure for the units with the blanket ban remaining as above, 0.023788, while the figure for the single ward, non-blanket policy units being 0.024485 fires per admission.

With a total of 65 fires reported, 35 (53.85%) were regarded as having been caused maliciously. If this figure is added to those for Self-harm, Suspicious and Unknown causes the total is 48 which is 73.85% of the reported fires.

Cigarettes, cigars and pipes proved to be the highest source of ignition with 24 incidents (36.9%) followed by lighters and then matches. In all, smokers materials accounted for 53 (81%) of the fires. Bedding (22 fires) followed by waste (18 fires) accounted for the material of first ignition for the majority of the fires.

Twenty three of the fires reported occurred in units with only one ward. The distribution of fires in larger units showed that the majority of fires, 59.5%, occurred on Rehabilitation and Pre-Discharge wards.

One unit provided results based on classifying one of their wards as both Admission and Intensive Care and the other as Rehabilitation/Pre-discharge. The combined figures for Intensive Care and Admission wards were a total of 11 fires (26%). Three fires (4.6%) occurred in areas common to all wards. Only one fire was reported from a ward providing a specialist treatment function, although this function was not defined by the respondent.

Bedrooms proved to be by far the major site for fires with 60% (39) of the incidents. Kitchens, day rooms and corridors or other circulation areas were far behind bedrooms with 8, 7 and 6 fires respectively. No fires were recorded in either offices or linen and other stores. Activity or Occupational Therapy rooms had two fires as did Bath and Clinic rooms. The majority of fires, 55 (86%), were classed as minor fires, meaning that they were, for example, extinguished by staff, caused little damage and no injury. The remainder of 9 fires (14%) were described as serious, eg., extinguished by the fire brigade, causing extensive damage or causing injury.

Discussion

The results showing the rates of fire per admission would appear to suggest that the use of blanket policies made no significant difference in reducing fire risk. Problems with the survey are of course that the sample is small (although unlikely to get much bigger!). In particular this may make the comparison of much more than the total figures meaningless. The results depend upon the honesty and accuracy of the respondents and their records. The sample itself could be biased in that those units which have responded may be aware that their record is particularly good.

The information requested was not detailed enough to allow any cross referencing to examine the effect that an 'epidemic' of fire setting or the behaviour of one particular patient might have on the results. Since only one of the small units reported a consistent ban policy no real comparison could be made between units of similar size.

Despite these criticisms and those of the figures taken from all the units without a total ban policy, these figures appear to be valid because they show what is to all intents and purposes an identical rate of fire.

Even if all of these units operated a system in which different wards operated different blanket policies this would still be seen to be at least as safe as banning matches and lighters totally

Taking the results from the single ward units without a ban policy, we still come up with a difference in the rate of fires per admission which is less than one fire per 1000 admissions. This would suggest that these units are at least as effective in reducing the risk of fire occurring as those units which ban the patients from having matches and lighters altogether.

In the units which allowed matches and lighters 59.4% of the fires were started with matches and lighters, cigarettes and other smokers materials for 28% and cookers for the remainder. The units operating a blanket policy showed matches and lighters at 27%, cigarettes and other smokers materials at 42% with cookers and other sources at 30%. While there is some difference in the figures for the two groups this shows that patients on the blanket ban policy units were still able to get matches and lighters to set fires with. This different pattern of fires is something which may reveal more information in future studies which are able to examine the records more closely. However the patients in the 'ban' units may have simply shifted to more easily accessible tools for their purpose.

The figures about the nature of the fires show that the majority of fires were set deliberately, and that cigarettes, pipes or cigars were the major source of ignition, although matches and lighters combined were greater still. Bedding followed by waste were the main materials ignited first and most fires started in bedrooms. Most fires were regarded as minor but a large minority were reported as being serious in nature. Most fires happened on wards which were described as having a rehabilitation function

Since the major fear usually expressed is about deliberate fire setting it is interesting to compare these figures with those from other hospitals. Stollard (1984), Chandler (1990) and Barker et al (1991) examined fire reports from the health service. Stollard examined results from one Regional Health Authority over several years, Chandler took figures from one year for all the hospitals in the UK. They showed respectively, figures of 25% and 19.5%, Chandler further analysed the figures and showed a rate for psychiatric hospitals of 35%. Barker et al (1991) found that in one psychiatric hospital 49% of fires were started deliberately while in the other the figure was 27%. This compares with a rate of 53% for fires identified as malicious in the Regional Secure Unit (RSU) sample. That figure does not include self-harm or suspicious causes which if included move the rate up to approximately 65%.

Given that it is possible that malicious fires in the Health service as a whole could be caused by outsiders as well as patients this shows quite a markedly increased rate of malicious firesetting in the RSU sample. Even given the slightly different classification system used this is an appreciable risk. Most modern RSU's are built with modern fire detection and prevention systems and have obviously more control over access by the public than the rest of the NHS.

Smokers' materials were the most important source of ignition in all studies. The other figures relating to the nature of the fires. show that in RSU's more fires occur in bedrooms than would be expected from the NHS figures. Bedding (34%), followed by waste (28%), becomes the highest risk material for first ignition. In a different study within the NHS the relative figures are 50% of fires started in waste and only 3.1% in bedding (Stollard 1983). This different pattern can possibly be accounted for by the prevalence of single bedrooms within the RSU's within which patients are usually allowed a fair amount of privacy.

No comparison could be obtained from the type of ward in which the fires started since this set-up is perhaps only repeated in some Psychiatric hospitals. However the figures do,suggest that the price of more liberal ward atmospheres on rehabilitation and pre-discharge areas is a slightly higher risk of fire. No information was requested which would show the comparative numbers of patients in the different areas. This would require further study since the information available does not allow that depth of analysis.

No information could be found that would allow for comparison of the rate of fire per admissions. Comments received from respondents showed that even amongst similar units which did not operate a blanket ban policy there were large differences in the way that the risk was managed. One unit banned matches because they were difficult to keep track of and would only allow staff to carry unit lighters. Another stuck to a totally individualised policy of only controlling access to these items with patients who were assessed to be of some risk. The involvement of patients by discussing the need to prevent a certain individual access to fire is something which might cause controversy amongst some nurses. The importance of individual assessments and programmes of supervised access and evaluation was emphasised by several respondents. One area which this author had not thought to examine was that of fires being set off the unit. One respondent reported as many fires being set in the main hospital by one or more of their patients as occurred on the unit.

Conclusion

The evidence from this survey suggests that there is a greater risk of deliberate firesetting on Regional Secure Units compared with other psychiatric and general hospitals in the National Health Service. The overall picture would suggest that the most common scenario for a fire on a Secure Unit would involve a patient using smokers' materials to set a fire to bedding in a bedroom on a Rehabilitation ward. This picture of deliberate fire setting as a likely problem on secure units reinforces the dilemma that nurses and other professionals face.

Many nurses working in this field may be familiar with a statement to the effect that 'We're in the risk game'. The measure of our success is probably in our ability to make the 'right' decisions which staff in other fields would not be happy making. The potential severity of a mistake made in our decisions enhances the perception of risk. As one respondent nearly put it 'All serious fires started off as minor ones.'

However the judgements about risk should be taken in the context of all the factors involved. If our role is to help our patients better their lives and protect the public at the same time can we do our job without taking some risks? How do we evaluate progress if we do not risk-take?

The literature offers little on which to base risk management of any kind in Regional Secure Units. The already published output on the service is mainly written from the medical model and does not discuss the dilemmas on the units themselves. However units have had to face these dilemmas and make decisions which may not have had any grounding in research. Nursing staff have the responsibility of managing the risk factors on a day to day basis (see DoH 1990 p79) and would seem to be the best placed to lead in the decision making.

The evidence from this survey would suggest that individualised forms of intervention are, in the case of fire risk, at least as effective as a blanket policy. The advantages in terms of a more 'normal' atmosphere for the majority of the patients and better chances for assessment and evaluation of firesetters would appear obvious and desirable. Regional Secure Units depend for their success on the building of trust between staff and patients. The fact that many of the patients will be allowed to leave the unit without escort shows that it is probably impossible to control the smuggling of banned items if the patient is determined enough.

Menzies (1959) argued that the rituals used by nurses to.defend against the anxieties of the job, were in fact ineffective and led to a decreased ability to cope with those anxieties. If the blanket policies were to be seen in a similar light, what is the effect on the staff of their lack of success?

Recommendations

More research needs to be carried out on the topic of fire risk management, which would probably involve a more in depth study of patient records and fire records to gain the necessary detail to cross reference the different factors. Since this survey used information which had been collected by the units for their own purposes and did not avail itself of any sophisticated analysis this can only be seen as a pointer to the need for future research. A fruitful avenue for research would appear to be comparing the practises of the different units in greater detail. Why do some units have low rates of fires whilst actually allowing patients to have lighters etc.? This could encompass the minutiae of how the policies are actually implemented and how patients are assessed. The model proposed by Jackson, Glass & Hope (1987) suggests that the person's situation has to be taken into account to understand the firesetting.

Another aspect which might be worthy of attention would be the effect of the social environment on the rate of fires. Are more restrictive units less able to meet the needs of the patients and therefore more likely to experience greater rates of firesetting or other destructive behaviours? Would research show higher rates of all destructive or disruptive behaviours?

Research into the knowledge, skills and attitudes which inform the decisions of staff in the secure units may provide information of value not only to other nurses and other disciplines but will help to raise the quality of care offered to our patients.

Nurses are the staff who have to deal daily with the problems of managing the risk on these units. It would therefore seem appropriate that they work to build a body of knowledge which will allow for decision making on the basis of predictable risk. The present picture suggests that, perhaps through no fault of individual nurses, this is more likely to be done on the basis of experience, anxiety or 'common sense'. To the present author this appears to be one of the major gaps in the repertoire of nursing in the Regional Secure Units

7 A view of seclusion in psychiatric nursing

Barry Topping-Morris

The humane treatment of the mentally ill has remained a sensitive issue ever since the time of the great Victorian reformers. Throughout the 1980's there was increased interest among Mental Health Service providers and the public in safeguarding civil and legal rights of mentally disordered patients. In focusing on the protection of the civil rights of patients many of the traditional aspects of mental health care have come to be challenged on their therapeutic as well as legal validity.

Seclusion, however, has managed to avoid the questioning eye of the mental health practitioner. Consequently, it has received very little attention in the literature. The aim of this chapter is to open up a needed dialogue amongst today's professionals on this common, albeit tyrannical, treatment relic of the past (Pillette 1978). The question posed is why seclusion still remains in the treatment repertoire of today's mental health care? This will be examined in the light of the recently published Code of Practice (1990), whose view is that seclusion is not a treatment technique and should not feature as part of any treatment programme.

The use of seclusion

The continued use of seclusion in psychiatry has been referred to as an embarrassing reality, and yet the practice continues. Is this because patients benefit, or is it because it is still easier to isolate an out of control patient behind a locked door than deal with the underlying problem (Hamil 1987)?

The frequency of use of seclusion varies in different hospitals and in-patient facilities, with the highest rate reported in locked short-term admission wards, where more than half the patients may be secluded at some stage of their stay. In less acute units, rates as low as 2 to 4% have been reported (Tardiff 1981).

The available studies generally indicate that secluded patients are predominantly young and have a diagnosis of schizophrenia or hypomanic illness, but the frequency of these diagnoses is in proportion with the frequency in the admission populations(Hodkinson 1985, Soloff 1983). Seclusion is most likely early in admission and is associated with a longer length of hospital stay (Soloff, Turner 1981). The duration of seclusion is variable, averages of one to two hours (Russell et al 1986), two hours (Morrison 1987), and ten hours (Soloff, Turner 1981) have been quoted in the available literature.

What is seclusion?

Definitions of seclusion range from the very simplistic to the elaborate. Campbell et al (1982) simply defines it as the act of temporarily isolating a disturbed patient in a locked room. The draft Code of Practice (DHSS 1983) painstakingly defines seclusion as 'the supervised confinement of a patient alone in a room which may be locked for the protection of others from significant harm, its sole aim therefore is to contain severely disturbed behaviour which is likely to cause harm to others. Seclusion is the supervised denial of the company of other people by constraint within a closed environment at any time of the day and night. The patient is confined alone in a room, the door of which cannot be unlocked from the inside, and from which there is no other means of exit open to the patient himself. Seclusion should always be distinguished from time out for positive reinforcement'.

Seclusion is commonly used in psychiatric nursing practice and the Royal College of Nursing (RCN 1979), in giving its guidelines on the issue, justifies its use as being 'necessary where there is an immediate danger to the patient or others'. This guidance may have indirectly resulted in the seclusion of numerous patients who have presented as being a danger to themselves when the depths of despair that these patients are experiencing warrant intensive specialised therapeutic intervention rather than a punitive custodial isolation. The Code of Practice thankfully recognises this more humanistic approach by adopting the stance that 'seclusion should never be used where there is a risk that the patient may take his own life or otherwise harm himself; its sole aim therefore is to contain severely disturbed behaviour which is likely to cause harm to others'.

The environment

To the inexperienced observer seclusion rooms look very frightening. They consist of a single room without furniture, except for a fixed bed and a mattress. The walls are bare, lighting is fixed to the ceiling, and a fixed opening with an unbreakable window is allowed for natural light and ventilation. The doors are reinforced, lockable, and have an integral unbreakable window for observational purposes (Macdonald 1988).

Conditions of seclusion were considered in the case of A v United Kingdom, which was considered by the European Commission of Human Rights (Bluglass and Bowden 1988). The case concerned a patient who was secluded in Broadmoor Hospital for five weeks in 1984, after being suspected of setting fire to a ward. It was claimed that the conditions in which he had been held, in a room with no furniture, daytime clothing or footwear, amounted to a breach of Article 3 of the European Convention on Human Rights, which prohibits 'torture or inhuman or degrading treatment or punishment' (Jacobs 1975). The Commission reached the provisional view that there had been a violation of Article 3, and it was accepted that the treatment could be degrading despite there being no intention to degrade. 'A friendly settlement' was reached between the parties, which included an undertaking to introduce written guidelines on the use of seclusion at Broadmoor Hospital. These make clear that the criterion for seclusion is the patient's own safety or that of others, and the guidelines specified conditions about space, lighting, clothing and other facilities.

Gibson (1989) and Campbell (1982) describe seclusion environments as being clinically cold and unwelcoming. Thankfully the modern stance being adopted by the Code of Practice recommends that seclusion should be in a safe, secure and properly identified room, where the patient cannot harm himself, accidentally or intentionally. The room should have adequate heating, light, ventilation and seating. The room should offer complete observation from the outside, while also affording the patient privacy from other patients.

Ethical and moral issues

An ethical dilemma arises when a nurse contemplates the use of seclusion (McCoy and Garritson 1983). It is where to draw the line between the infringement of personal liberty for a difficult or potentially dangerous patient and the probable benefits of the other patients on the ward from that infringement. Pilette (1978) strongly objects to decisions on seclusion being made on this basis. She comments that in such a utilitarian approach essentially anything that disturbs the tranquillity of the mental ward is punishable by seclusion. Morrison (1987) considered seclusion to be associated more with the traditional custodian mode of psychiatric nursing than with current nursing ideologies. The RCN Society of Psychiatric Nursing (1979) firmly believed that seclusion should only be used when other means to try to contain a situation had been exhausted, but recognised that, particularly because of staff shortages, it may from time to time be a necessary procedure. This stance begs the question, is it just to inflict such punishment on an individual, who is without crime or trial, in the name of treatment and the welfare of the community (Pillette 1978).

Whilst the RCN guidelines condone the use of seclusion as a necessary procedure, particularly because of staff shortages, the Code of Practice suggests 'its use cannot be foreseen, it should not be used because of staff shortages'. Gibson (1989) remarks that; if one accepts that the use of seclusion is largely determined by staff levels, then one must accept that this is a misuse of seclusion as the client would not need the intervention of seclusion if staffing levels were satisfactory.

MP

Discussion

Whilst seclusion may occasionally be necessary, its over use can also be a sensitive indicator of poor practice and staff difficulties in hospitals, and the practice therefore requires strict guidelines and external monitoring. Despite this, neither the 1959 nor the 1983 Mental Health Acts mention seclusion. In the latter case this was probably a deliberate omission to allow the newly formed Mental Health Act Commission an opportunity to examine and prepare guidance on the issue (Leopold 1985). The legal justification for seclusion concerns the right to restrain a patient who is doing, or is about to do, physical harm to himself, to another person or to property.

However, the decision to seclude a patient is frequently based upon the utilitarian rule which is fashioned to yield the greatest tranquillity or the least unhappiness for the rest of the patients and staff. Seclusion is a method of control that is employed to protect patients from themselves and others from them. This most inhumane cruelty of man to man can become routine if it is surrounded and buffered by the facade of being 'therapeutic'. Seclusion ignores and devalues the most basic quality of man - his choice. If anything, it encourages regressive choices, a falling away from full humanness and further loss of control. Seclusion does do its protective job well for staff and other patients but at the expense of marking the secluded individual with psychic wounds far deeper than any that may be averted. It also takes the individual farther than ever away from inner tranquillity and control. O'Gorman (1976) suggests that not enough emphasis is given to the preventative aspects of caring for people who become disturbed, the implication being that much disturbed behaviour, and the seclusion used to contain it, could be reduced through adequate programmes of rehabilitation and occupation. Campbell (1982) found that nursing attitudes towards the use of seclusion varied a good deal according to the individual nurse. He also found that nursing staff in particular had learned a good deal from close examinations of their feelings towards aggressive patients. Whereas generally we feel it is too much to ask nurses never to feel anger towards a difficult patient, it is essential that such feelings should be recognised by the team as a whole. If this is not done, then the dangers are that staff aggression may be 'acted out', perhaps unconsciously.

The way forward

Clearly, critical evaluation and a careful weighing of the pros and cons of seclusion are required of us. As patient advocates we must open up and air the issue of seclusion; exposing it as a lingering relic of the past. Such action is not simply a matter of safeguarding patients' civil rights but a matter of guaranteeing their human rights as well.

For reforms to take place attitudes need to be changed. It is necessary to increase nurses sensitivity and self awareness regarding the use of seclusion. Time should be devoted to experiential learning. Clients views should also be included in the statutory procedure for seclusion, thus promoting discussion between the client and the nurse. These steps would add a more humane dimension to the use of seclusion (1989). In addition, staffing levels should be kept at an adequate level. If a client needs the intervention of seclusion largely because of poor staffing, a written report of this should be included in the reasons for seclusion.

MacDonald (1988) suggests that nursing teams should discuss the situation concerning seclusion and record their comments. This would enable the creation of a learning situation, where all staff would benefit from critical appraisal of the incident and therefore be able to map out strategies for preventing any similar occurrences in the future. It is also thought necessary to develop the team approach and to improve individual skills through peer group advice. Debriefing sessions prove exceptionally valuable in skills and attitudinal development. All this would ensure that the likelihood of seclusion is further reduced and a far more positive climate is widespread.

What needs to be done to improve the situation? We need to prevent services from using seclusion as a necessary leverage of control over the acting out of patients. We need to discourage the belief that human beings deserve inhumane treatment, that they can be treated without choice. To prevent the patient remaining in oppression we must remove the inclination for nursing staff to exercise control over patients and replace this with the nurses desire to teach patients how to control themselves.

In this regard, the message from the Code of Practice is very clear and is enshrined within its broad principles; 'patients should be delivered any necessary treatment or care in the least controlled and segregated facilities practicable'. The onus now rests with the practitioner and his/her ability to reflect the goodwill of the Code in the good practice offered to patients presenting with particular management problems.

8 Evaluating the preparation of forensic psychiatric nurses

Neil Kitchiner and Paul Rogers

Many of the chapters in this book have highlighted the need for formal training in a variety of aspects of the forensic psychiatric nursing field. This chapters offers the findings of a small, evaluative study of some nurses responses to a training initiative within a new forensic setting.

The Caswell Clinic is the first secure unit to open as part of the Mental Illness Services 'A Strategy for Wales' (Welsh Office May 1989). The clinic has a capacity to accept eighteen patients who require medium levels of security. The beds are divided between two wards, six beds make up the intensive care unit (ICU), the philosophy of which is to provide an environment which allows for an in depth assessment and or treatment for varying degrees of difficult behaviour. The remaining twelve beds make up the rehabilitation ward, the principle role is to provide the main base for treatment and rehabilitation, of those patients, who do not require the intensive nursing care and supervision provided by the intensive care\assessment ward. With the eventual aim of helping the patient to return to live in the community or a less secure setting.

Prior to the opening of the ISU, all the nursing staff underwent a seven week induction period. It's aim to update existing knowledge, skills, providing an insight into the philosophy and new skills required to work within a secure environment.   The planned programme of induction consisted of:

- Outside speakers providing information on their sphere of operations within forensic psychiatry i.e MIND, and WISH (Women in Special Hospitals and Secure Units).

- Internal speakers, who form part of the new service i.e. the role of the responsible medical officer, the forensic clinical psychologist, the occupational therapist, social workers etc.

- Areas covered within the induction were :- workshops on the management of violence, various team building sessions both formally and informally and an eight day control and restraint training course, which was attended by eighteen members of the thirty six staff group.

- Staff were also given the opportunity of visiting other controlled environments, which provide security for the mentally disordered offenders. These included special hospitals, regional secure units, and HM Prisons.

- Some nursing staff had the opportunity to take part in nursing assessments under supervision of more experienced staff, of those patients detained in the above environments who had been referred to the clinic for possible admission.

- From day one of the induction the staff group were divided into seven small groups consisting of five to six nurses. Each group comprised of an F grade charge nurse who adopted the role of team leader, E and D grade staff nurses, D grade enrolled nurses and A grade care assistants.

These groups provided a forum in which staff could start to develop closer relationships with each other, critique operational policies and work on various small self directed projects which were presented to all the staff at the end of the induction.

During the seven weeks induction family and staff social events were encouraged, resulting in two social evenings, one which took place on the unit, the other at a local social club.

Background

A review of the literature yielded very little information on previous work in this area. Forensic psychiatric nursing in England has been described as a speciality (Parry 1991 and Pendersen 1988), most often because of the secure nature of the care environments, the potential dangerousness of clients and the relationship of the offence with the presenting mental illness.

If forensic nursing is deemed a speciality within psychiatry, then it would seem appropriate that the nurse entering this field of nursing, should be equipped with specialist skills and knowledge. This view is endorsed by Gostin (1985), who recommends that to have as few non physical aspects of security, dependant upon the skills and attitudes of the staff employed to work within these secure units.

There is very little literature available on forensic nursing skills, apart from a study by Phillips (1980 and 1983) who looked into the training needs of the Canadian forensic nurses. He described the development of a programme that had a `forensic module', available as part of an advanced psychiatric nursing certificate.

It is interesting to note from Phillips' study (1983), that the impression that forensic nursing does not require a specialist training, that in fact advancement of skills generally would improve services. This point was again emphasised when 80% of nationally surveyed forensic and generic psychiatric nurses felt that all mental health disciplines needed post graduate training in forensic client care. This suggests no specialist skills or knowledge are accredited to or needed by forensic nurses.

Niskala (1986) contradicts the above, she asserts from her research into 'competencies and skills required by nurses working in forensic areas', that many forensic nurses express the belief that there are certain areas within forensic nursing that require special skills i.e. maintaining security and instructing offenders.

A recent study by Kitchiner et al (1992), looked at `the role of the forensic psychiatric nurse' in England and Wales. The study highlighted the important issues identified by forensic psychiatric nurses currently employed in practice. These fell into two major categories : those concerned with therapy and those concerned with control. For example, 86% of respondents felt forensic nurses should be self aware, 79% felt they should be able to communicate effectively with others and 78% felt they should be able to develop close therapeutic relationships (therapy issues). On the other hand, 84% felt forensic psychiatric nurses should have a knowledge of assessing dangerousness, 76% felt they should be able to handle violence and 69% felt they should be able to demonstrate an ability to deal with hostility.

In England, the English National Board has recently approved the second generation of courses aimed at psychiatric nurse practitioners, working in controlled environments (E.N.B. 770). This course is intended to develop the specialism (forensic nursing), by creating a body of knowledge and enhancing the quality of nursing offered to patients (Tarbuck 1990).

It is currently the only course offered to nurses working within controlled environments and is only available in a handful of places in England at present. The course varies from place to place, in some regions it is full time, lasting nine months, in others it is only for six months, at present there are plans to make it available as a distanced learning package to ease the burden on managers losing staff for such long periods.

This type of course will go some way to addressing the many issues with which the nurse comes up against when working in this area. As yet there is no recognised course available to the unqualified nurse (care assistants). Their needs are often not catered for when reviewing the training needs of a staff group. Yet they are expected to take on many responsibilities with little or no formal training. As a new service is developed to meet the needs of it's intended population and catchment area, it brings with it many new job opportunities, right across the spectrum of mental health care professionals. In nursing terms we can expect to see recruitment from all the grades, from the care assistant (grade A) to the clinical nurse manager (grade I). This new skill mix will comprise of individuals with varying ages, gender, personal life experiences, ethnicity, etc, into one controlled environment.

Forgas (1985) writes about the process of becoming acquainted with a group of strangers and forming a new social unit, a group, out of a collection of individuals and how this places special strains on most peoples interactive skills. This problem is not a new one, it has been a major factor in staff recruitment for many years, the 1950's saw the use of behavioural science theories, steadily incorporated into personnel departments. Staff development at the place of work is usually concerned either with helping individuals settle into a new job or with helping those in the job to do that job more effectively and efficiently. Hunter and Russel (1990), wrote about the process of staff induction programmes being concerned with people settling in to their new surroundings as quickly as possible and for them to become fully productive without delay. Staff training is likely to be effective, depending on the relevance of what is ordered and also on the training techniques employed.

Aims of the study

The aim of the study was to assess and evaluate how prepared the staff group felt following a seven week induction period and to identify any anxieties which may be present.

Sample

The sample consisted of all thirty six nursing staff, of grades A to I, recently recruited to work within the Caswell Clinic interim secure unit, Glanrhyd hospital, Bridgend, Mid-Glamorgan.

Methodology

The collection of data was collected via a simple questionnaire. Information collected included:

- personnel details, name (optional), grade, gender, qualified\unqualified, name of ward and any previous experience of working within a secure setting;

- a list of how prepared or not prepared each respondent felt for the opening of the unit.

The questionnaire was then circulated to all grades of the units nursing staff, with an attached letter explaining the outline and aim of the study. Over a period of two weeks, the staff were given three reminders to complete and return the questionnaires. The data collected was then analysed and put into different sub groups, allowing for comparisons and to highlight any trends.

Findings

The returned questionnaires totalled thirty six completed replies, making a 100% return rate.

Table 1 Profile of the sample

Job title	Grade	Number	% of total staff group
Care assistant	A	7	19.4
Enrolled nurse	D	4	11.1
Staff nurse	D	10	27.7
Staff nurse	E	7	19.4
Charge nurse	F	5	13.8
Ward manager	G	2	5.4
Clinical nurse manager	I	1	2.7

The staff gender results showed a total of 15 (41.5%) were male and 21 (58.8%) were female. Qualified nurses represented the highest percentage of staff (80%). The remaining (20%) were care assistants (unqualified). Ward placement showed a distribution of (42%) working in ICU and (56%) working on the rehabilitation ward. Numbers of staff who had previous experience of working within controlled environments was relatively low only (17%), the remaining (83%) had no previous experience of controlled environments.

The thirty six respondents offered a total of 250 items describing factors that were to do with whether or not staff felt prepared to work in the new forensic unit. Thirty three respondents identified both positive and negative factors. Three respondents offered only factors that contributed to their feeling prepared In total 66% of the factors identified were positive and 34% were negative.

A more in depth breakdown with examples of the items given by each grade are as follows.

Grade A (care assistants)

Factors that contributed to respondents' feeling prepared were:- the induction, team building exercises, control and restraint training and approachable management.

Factors that contributed to respondents' feeling unprepared were:- a need for more input into the practical aspects of forensic nursing i.e. use of special observations, counselling skills and a greater knowledge of medication and it's effects.

Grade D (enrolled nurses)

Factors that contributed to respondents' feeling prepared were:- the induction, team building exercises, control and restraint training, exposure to the client group through assessments and patient profiles prior to admission.

Factors that contributed to respondents' feeling unprepared were:- a need for a greater emphasis in the practical procedures i.e. fire drills, how to observe patients, uncertainties regarding the enrolled nurses position within the staff team.

Grade D (staff nurses)

Factors that contributed to respondents' feeling prepared were:- previous experience within generic psychiatry including RMN training, confidence in the new nursing team, induction and approachable management.

Factors that contributed to respondents' feeling unprepared were:- uncertainty about the role of the D grade staff nurse, lack of previous forensic experience, uncertainty about practical skills i.e. ordering of ward supplies and fire drills.

Grade E (staff nurses)

Factors that contributed to respondents' feeling prepared were:- induction, team building exercises, past experience within generic psychiatry and the patient profiles prior to admission.

Factors that contributed to respondents' feeling unprepared were:- no previous experience in forensic psychiatry, unsure of role, lack of knowledge regarding part III of mental health act 1983, practical skills i.e day to day management of the ward.

Grade F (charge nurses)

Factors that contributed to respondents' feeling prepared were:- previous experience within forensic nursing and RMN training, attending the ENB 770 course and other post registration courses, induction, team building, previous generic experience.

Factors that contributed to respondents' feeling unprepared were:- unsure of new role, management issues, lack of practical skills i.e. patient assessments, part III of the mental health act, anxieties that not all staff had been trained in control and restraint techniques.

Grade G (ward managers and grade I clinical nurse manager)

Factors that contributed to respondents' feeling prepared were:- All had previous forensic experience, RMN training and ENB 770 course, personal attributes i.e confidence and flexibility.

Factors that contributed to respondents' feeling unprepared were:- new role, ward systems, i.e paper work, communication channels not fully established and lack of forensic experience in new work force.

Discussion

On examination of the main themes, there appears to be very little difference between the factors that contributed to respondents' feeling prepared for the A grade care assistants and the F grade charge nurses. However the factors that contributed to respondents' feeling unprepared demonstrate that the A grades require further practical input, whilst the F grade nurses main reasons for feeling unprepared was as a direct result of their new role.

It is interesting to note that the F grades reasons were not entirely directed at their own individual needs but also at the needs of the service i.e. lack of assessment tools, only half the staff had been trained in control and restraint techniques. This appears to demonstrates a consideration of the ward management issues which their new role will require.

On the whole, the nursing staff felt prepared (66%) for the opening of the unit, the common most reasons that emerge across all grades of staff for this preparedness are:- the induction programme, team building exercises, control and restraint techniques, approachable and experienced senior nursing staff and the opportunity to undertake patient assessments prior to the unit opening.

The main reasons why staff appeared to feel unprepared relate to uncertainties and anxieties about their new role. Kitchiner et al (1992), identified that role conflict and role ambiguity are common problems facing forensic nurses and that forensic nurses see their role as both controlling and therapeutic. The remaining reasons for unpreparedness to emerge were:- a lack of forensic nursing experience, uncertainty about ward systems and practical day to day management issues relating to the forensic patient.

Conclusions, limitations and recommendations for further study

The results seem to indicate that a planned induction for newly appointed staff, who are entering a work place in which they have very little experience, will aid to help them to settle in more quickly and feel comfortable with their new role. The authors put forward the following recommendations for those managers in the future who might run a similar induction programme for newly appointed nurses coming to work within a controlled environment.

- Induction courses should wherever possible address the individuals needs more closely, rather than those of the group or organisations.

- There should be an ongoing evaluation of the induction programme from day one, with the provision to change the programme around to meet the needs of the staff being inducted, to remain flexible.

- Induction programmes should have a balance between theoretical and skills based components.

- Induction programmes should be planned with enough time for new staff to do at least one working placement, within a controlled environment as similar to their own place of work. So that they may gain insight and experience into an established forensic setting and to help relieve any anxieties they may have.

- Unqualified staff need more practical input which will help them with their new role and less theoretical knowledge.

- At the end of any induction programme nurses should be encouraged to voice unprepared feelings to their superiors. With the view that areas of unpreparedness can be swiftly addressed.

A further evaluation should take place after six months, allowing for a comparison of the results and to highlight any areas of unpreparedness amongst staff.

9 The expanded role of the forensic psychiatric nurse

Philip Burnard

The role of the forensic psychiatric nurse is an complex one. As we have seen in this book, people who look after forensic psychiatric patients may be called nurses, prison officers, clinical nurse specialists or forensic clinical nurse specialists. The people for whom they care may be referred to as patients, clients, inmates or prisoners. Forensic psychiatric nursing seems to be concerned with a range of things that are outside of the usual remit of nursing. The forensic nurse will be forced to consider illness, crime, morality, treatment, containment and possibly punishment. Within this complicated and sometimes contradictory picture arises the question of the *role* of the forensic psychiatric nurse.

What might be the aim of forensic psychiatric nursing? It is to help in the 'recovery' of 'patients' or is it the containment of those who are deemed to have broken the law and who happen, also, to be mentally ill? Clearly, the two issues are not exclusive. It is possible to adopt a position in which it is felt that the law has been broken by a person who is mentally ill and that help in healing the mental illness may prevent recidivism in the future. All of this presupposes that the terms 'mentally ill', 'treatment' and 'healing' are clear cut: clearly, they are not. It is by no means established that certain mental illnesses deem some people more likely to break the law. Nor has it been established that 'therapy', in any sense at all, is guaranteed to prevent recidivism.

Nor has it even been established that treatments of mental illness are particularly effective. Thus, the forensic psychiatric nurse is caught up in a role that contains a number of facets, some of which appear to be contradictory and in which they are being asked to be therapist and agent of social control.

Two elements of the role of the forensic nurse have been discussed at various points in this book. Many forensic psychiatric nurses appear to view their role as involving both a *therapeutic* and a *security* role. At first glance, the two elements seems to illustrate the contradiction in the role of the nurse in its most extreme form. Most of the writers on psychotherapy have stressed the need for a *voluntary* relationship between therapist and client. Clearly, too, it would seem to be unlikely that anyone could insist that another person received therapy - at least, therapy that was likely to be beneficial. The nurse, therefore, finds him or herself in the position of insisting that he or she contains the client but, is also wanting to offer help and therapy.

Murray Cox (1990), sometime psychotherapist at Broadmoor hospital suggests that there need be no contradiction here. He suggests that once the client has acknowledge the limitations that have necessarily been imposed on him or her, he or she can open up to the possibility of therapy. In a sense, of course, everyone who receives therapy is constrained. No one has complete freedom. We all live in a world were what we would like to do has to be compared with what we are free to do. All therapy must acknowledge the limitations of the client's life world and must remain 'practical'. In this sense, the person who finds him or herself in a forensic unit, a psychiatric unit in a prison or in a special hospital is in the extreme position of the one that we all experience in a rather less extreme way. In fact, the 'containment' element of being in a forensic unit can, paradoxically, be liberating. Let us consider this view a little further.

First, unlike most other people who receive therapy, the forensic client or patient is, like all his colleagues, *necessarily* constrained. This is not generally true of the psychiatric patient in a general psychiatric unit or hospital. The vast majority of people in psychiatric hospitals are free to leave. The patient or client in a forensic unit is, most definitely, not. Thus, those people who are receiving therapy in a forensic setting are all experiencing similar living conditions. Whilst their perception of those conditions will vary, the fact that they are all in a similar situation means that they have, at once, one thing in common. This, in itself, can enable a sense of community to be developed in, for example, group therapy. Given that the nurses in such settings are also sharing a considerable amount of the client's life world, they, too, seem ideally placed to work in therapeutic ways. On the other hand, it may be noted that this idea of a 'therapeutic role' has not been discussed, in great length, in this book. It would appear that forensic psychiatric nurses may still have to develop this therapeutic element of their work.

Second, the fact that in any forensic setting there are people who live together and who are bound to do so, means that no one can easily remove themselves from the therapeutic environment, once they are committed to it. This might work in one of two ways. It might, on the one hand, cause 'therapeutic claustrophobia' - a 'hothouse' atmosphere where everyone feels that every aspect of their lives are constantly under review. On the other hand, it might enable deeper therapeutic work to be carried out, in the style of intensive workshops and therapy sessions that take place away from forensic settings. The closed world of the forensic unit may offer just the right environment for intensive therapy. All of this would, of course, have to be predicated on the idea that the clients have, in Cox's sense, accepted the limitations of their confinement.

If this therapeutic atmosphere is to flourish, it seems likely that the nurses who work in such units are going to have to review their roles in fairly considerably. Often, the ethos in special hospitals, prisons and some forensic units encourages and emphasis on containment. There is, in such institutions, a clear demarcation between 'staff' and 'patients'. Goffman (1961) identified this separation of roles and of worlds in his study of 'total institutions'. Indeed, one of the factors that makes a total institution 'work' is just this separation of roles. On the other hand, part of being a therapist involves a blurring of roles between clients and therapists. Therapy may involve self-disclosure on the part of the therapist as well as on the part of the client (Burnard and Morrison 1992). The change of role, then, would not only be an organisational one, but also a personal one.

Next, nurses who worked in therapeutic ways would need support. Much has been written about the need for therapists and counsellors to work under supervision (Hawkins and Shoet 1989). Most people who listen to the pains and problems of other people need to be able to offload and to discuss progress of lack of it. One of the idiosyncratic factors about such supervision, within forensic settings, would be that the supervisor would also have to be a member of the same community. Given the fact that all information about patients and clients in forensic settings is confidential and that in most units, the staff are bound by the Official Secrets Act, the idea of bringing in a supervisor from outside of the organisation would seem to be ruled out. Also, staff would have to acknowledge the *need* for such supervision.

Finally, in this short consideration of some of the therapeutic elements of the role of the forensic nurse, comes the issues of training. The 1982 syllabus of training for psychiatric nurses differed from all previous syllabi in its accent on psychiatric nursing skills of a therapeutic nature. The training courses that followed the publication of that syllabus emphasised the need for helping psychiatric nurses to develop self-awareness and counselling skills. Since the publication of that syllabus, there have been many publications on the topic of training nurses in such therapeutic skills (Burnard 1990).

The forensic nurse as counsellor

Whilst full psychotherapy may or may not be outside of the role of the forensic psychiatric nurse, most qualified forensic nurses might consider counselling as part of what they do. In this final section, the notion of counselling within forensic nursing is briefly explored.

What is counselling?

Counselling is something that most forensic nurses do, formally or informally. It is probably what everyone does. Right from the start, it is important to demystify the process for if we do not, there is a danger that we might miss some important chances to help others.

Counselling has been defined in many ways in many books. Most definitions offer variations around the following key points : counselling involves:

- two people, one of whom is identified as a counsellor and the other who can be called the client;

- the helping of the client by the counsellor;

- a situation in which the client has problems, sometimes clearly identify and sometimes not, which he or she shares with the counsellor;

- a relationship that is different to plain 'conversation' and yet is not psychotherapy.

What is a therapeutic relationship?

We all have a variety of relationships with a variety of different people. We may have formal, work-related relationships with colleagues, for example. We have closer relationship and of a different sort, with parents and members of the family. We have relationships that are closer still, and yet different again, with friends and those with whom we fall in love.

I am using the term 'therapeutic relationship' to describe the sort of relationship that occurs in counselling. There is no doubt that the relationship is central to counselling. Patterson says this on the subject:

> Counselling or psychotherapy is an interpersonal relationship. Note that I don't say that counselling or psychotherapy involves and interpersonal relationship - it is an interpersonal relationship (Patterson 1985).

The therapeutic relationship is almost paradoxical for it is close and yet professional. It is warm and genuine and yet you don't fall in love with the other person. You care for them and yet not in the way that you do about your family. Most of all, the therapeutic relationship is a helping relationship in which the person who is the counsellor is helping the person called the client.

Of course, it is not always as simple as this. We are often helped by our clients. We often learn as much about ourselves when we do

143

counselling as we do about the other person. But the point is that the counsellors intention in counselling is to be helpful and thus therapeutic for the other person. You do not set out in counselling to sort out your own problems. You do not set out in counselling to sort out the other person's problems either but you do start with the aim of helping the other person in their struggle. This, then, is the therapeutic relationship. It can be characterised in the following ways :

- there is an intention on the part of the counsellor to help;

- the relationship is of benefit to the client;

- the counsellor cares about the client;

- the relationship is reciprocated to some degree but, in the end, it is the client's needs who are uppermost;

- the relationship is always an ethical one and is not exploited by the counsellor.

The last two issues are vital. Not all therapeutic relationships are necessarily reciprocal ones. That is to say that it is not always the case that the counsellor and client both feel close to one another. Certainly, the pair do not share all of their problems in a reciprocal way.

Also, the relationship is bound to be an ethical one. The client must be able to trust the counsellor and the counsellor must always act as a professional person. After all, the client is sharing important and personal information with the counsellor and a close relationship often results from this sharing. It is essential, if the relationship is to remain therapeutic (and not become some other sort of relationship) that the counsellor always acts in the best interests of the client and according to that person's wishes.

Counselling and psychotherapy

Psychotherapy is an umbrella term for a wide range of therapies that are usually used to help people who are suffering from mental ill health, who want to solve some fairly deep seated personal problems or who feel that they want to develop themselves through a therapeutic relationship. Examples of the varieties of psychotherapy include (amongst others):

- *Psychoanalysis*. This well-known but less practiced therapy is based on the work of Freud. It is usually a lengthy therapy and, thus, necessarily costly. It is rarely available as a treatment within the National Health Service except in specialist units.

- *Behaviour therapy*. Popular for a considerable time with specially trained psychiatric nurses, behaviour therapy works at the level of attempting to change behaviour through schedules of reinforcement.

- *Gestalt therapy*. An 'alternative' therapy, based on the original work of Fritz Perls, gestalt therapy combines aspects of psychoanalysis with Oriental philosophy and a large element of the '60's 'here and now' approach to working with thoughts and feelings.

- *Transactional analysis*. A neo-Freudian therapy, developed by Eric Berne, transactional analysis works on the principle that everyone has three potential ego states: a parent, adult and child. It works by helping people to recognise certain patterns of behaviour within these ego stages.

- *Group therapy*. An economical approach to therapy, the group approach can be conducted from a range of different theoretical viewpoints.

Normally, a psychotherapist has had a fairly lengthy and intense training. Most psychotherapists have also been in therapy themselves as this is considered necessary for the development of the personal and technical skills required to be a therapist. It is suggested, here, that the notion of counselling as part of the forensic psychiatric nurses' role seems more appropriate than that of psychotherapy.

145

Another way of looking at the differences between psychotherapy and counselling is to consider that psychotherapy is a much 'heavier' sort of process than is counselling. That is to say that the psychotherapist encourages the client to dig deeper into his or her feelings than is usually the case in counselling and to explore the client's world in much more detail.

Whilst the sort of counselling advocated for forensic nurses also takes into account the client's feelings, the idea of in depth exploration of this sort is not discussed. Any nurse who wants to take up psychotherapy should consider formal training. Oddly, though, no one has to train as a psychotherapist in order to call themselves one. That has led to a few people undertaking very short trainings and then practising as psychotherapists. It would be hard to justify this sort of approach, given the fragility of other human beings. Anyone seeking psychotherapy would be well advised to check the credentials and training of the person offering therapy.

Should all forensic nurses counsel?

Probably. As we noted above, the role of the forensic nurse is changing. Project 2000 courses have reflected the changing role of the nurse. Primary nursing, nursing theory and the social sciences literature all stress the need for forensic nurses to care for the whole person : emotional stresses and all. If we are to function as people who care for the whole person, we need to develop those specific skills to do the job.

Some will say that they don't need training: they are 'naturally' good at talking to people. No doubt this is true of some people. The point is that counselling is less about talking to people and much more about listening. Throughout this book and at the risk of becoming boring, the emphasis will be on developing listening skills. It is only when we can walk beside the other person, enter their world-view and understand things the way that they understand things that we will begin to become effective as counsellors. Listening, then, is the key skill in counselling. We all learned to listen in the first place. We can all learn to do it better.

All this is not to suggest that counselling is all that forensic nurses will do. It is not being advocated that forensic nurses be forced to set themselves up as general counsellors and offer help on all sorts of psychological matters. It is merely to note that the sorts of skills that can safely be called 'counselling skills' are useful to all forensic nurses in all aspects of his or her work. Counselling skills can enhance communication and caring between forensic nurses and patients, nurses and nurses and nurses and other sorts of colleagues.

In the end, too, they can help us to sort out some of our own problems. For in the end, we are also fragile and in need of help. As obvious as this seems now, it is not so long ago that forensic nurses were expected to be devoid of emotions and devoid of problems. The 'stiff upper lip' was the norm and if you had feelings you were expected to hide them. The atmosphere in nursing is changing. Slowly it is being recognised that we are all human and that we all suffer to some degree. Counselling skills can help to make us more human, more caring and more able to care. For it is one thing to intend to care and quite another to have the practical skills to be able to care.

Forensic nurses and counselling

There is not a long tradition of forensic nurses as counsellors. Nor do forensic nurses necessarily see themselves as fitting into the role of the counsellor. In a recent study of nurses attitudes towards counselling skills, we found that most nurses tended towards advice giving and prescription rather than towards listening and encouraging (Burnard and Morrison 1987). In another study, we found that nurses thought themselves far more able to given information and advice than to handle feelings and confrontation (Burnard and Morrison 1989).

It is suggested that counselling is much more about listening, encouraging and caring than it is about giving advice and information. Sometimes , of course, it will be necessary to give advice and information. This is rarely the case when it comes to personal problems and feelings. In the domain of my problems and feelings, I am the expert. It would be odd to argue otherwise. Could anyone really claim to know what is best for me? Would you like it if someone claimed to know what was best for you? I doubt it. And yet, up and down the country, it is still possible to hear people say things like : 'If I were you, I would ...' or 'Well, you know what you have to do now. You have to...' The implication is that it is possible to be an expert for someone else. This implication is the one that is challenged most strongly in this book. If we want our clients to develop autonomy and personal strength, then we must trust them to be the authority on their own lives.

Basic principles of counselling

From the discussion, above, it is possible to draw out some basic principles of counselling in nursing and ones that are applicable to forensic nursing. The list, below, is not an exhaustive one. It does not cover every possible principle of counselling. It is offered more as a basis for introducing the topic and for discussion.

● The client knows best. He or she is the expert on his or her problems and feelings. In the end, only he or she can make decisions about them. This would seem to apply just as much to forensic clients as to any other. The critical issue, here, is the degree to which people might *trust* that the client 'knows best' and the degree to which such knowledge might be acted upon.

● Interpretation by another person rarely helps. That is to say that it rarely helps to say things like 'What you really mean is...' or 'I know you think that's true but what is really happening is...' It seems to the editors that psychiatry is often based on interpretations of client behaviour. Another approach might be to attempt to remain at the level of *description* for as long as possible in the belief that sufficient description will offer the development of a much more thoroughgoing theory. Too often, it seems to us, health care professionals are tempted to rush in with spurious interpretations based on a less than thorough understanding of the psychological theory behind those interpretations - a sort of 'professional armchair philosophising'.

● It is important to enter the client's 'frame of reference'. We all look at the world in a unique sort of way. If we are to begin to understand the other person and to help them, it is vital that we try to view the world as they do. Entering the frame of reference of a forensic client, may, on occasions, be difficult. Also, entering the frame of reference of the client may require a radical shift of role on the part of some forensic professionals. It necessarily involves the health professional dropping some 'professionalism' and being prepared to meet the other person head on - as another human being. As Martin Buber had it, the 'I-Thou' relationship, rather than the 'I-It' relationship. In the 'I-Thou' relationship, both professional and client remain subjects. In the 'I-It' relationship, the professional, through distance, turns the client into an 'object' which, in turn, allows him or her to treat the client in a particular sort of way and to rationalise and justify behaviour that he or she would not justify if the relationship remained an 'I-Thou' one.

- Judgement and moralising are rarely appropriate. What has happened has happened. It is rarely helpful to blame the client or to say 'I'm not surprise at what has happened...why ever did you do that in the first place?' This would seem to be a particularly important issue in the field of forensic nursing. It is to be imagined that the judgement and moralisation has already taken place once a client enters a forensic psychiatric unit.

- Your experience is not the same as the clients's. This really is a fundamental rule. It is very easy to for me to begin to compare my life with yours or my experience with your experience. And yet we both have different histories and look at things from different points of view. Therefore, be very careful before you say things like : 'I know just what you mean...I'm just like that myself'. One thing is for sure : you are not. This may be even more evident in the field of forensic psychiatry.

- Listening is the first and last principle of good counselling. There need be no qualification of this principle. Whatever the context, forensic or otherwise, listening remains the basic ingredient of effective counselling.

Types of counselling

Client centred counselling

Whilst there are numerous approaches to counselling, client-centred counselling is probably the most widely known type of counselling and possibly the most widely used. The term 'client-centred', first used by Carl Rogers (1964) refers to the notion that it is the client, himself, who is best able to decide how to find the solutions to their problems in living. 'Client-centred', in this sense may be contrasted with the idea of 'counsellor-centred' or 'professional-centred', both of which may suggest that someone other than the client is the 'expert'. Whilst this may be true when applied to certain concrete 'factual' problems : housing, surgery, legal problems and so forth, it is difficult to see how it can apply to personal life issues. In such cases, it is the client who identifies the problem and the client who, given time and space, can find their way through the problem to the solution.

Client-centred counselling is a process rather than a particular set of skills. It evolves through the relationship that the counsellor has with the client and vice versa. In a sense, it is a period of growth for both parties, for both learns from the other. It also involves the exercise of restraint. The counsellor must restrain herself from offering advice and from the temptation to 'put the client's life right for him. The outcome of such counselling cannot be predicted nor can concrete goals be set (unless they are devised by the client, at their request). In essence, client-centred counselling involves an act of faith : a belief in the other person's ability to find solutions through the process of therapeutic conversation and through the act of being engaged in a close relationship with another human being.

Certain, basic client-centred skills may be identified, although as we have noted, it is the total relationship that is important. Skills exercised in isolation amount to little : the warmth, genuineness and positive regard must also be present. On the other hand, if basic skills are not considered, then the counselling process will probably be shapeless or it will degenerate into the counsellor becoming prescriptive. The skill of standing back and allowing the client to find his own way is a difficult one to learn.

We may well find that the client-centred approach to counselling is linked to a particular period of history - the middle of the 20th century. What characterises the client centred approach more than anything is the emphasis on the idea that the client is necessarily the person to sort out his or her own problems. Autonomy and freedom to choose are hallmarks of this approach. It is here that a curious paradox occurs. The one thing that forensic clients do not have is actual freedom. They do, in the existential sense, however, have a degree of mental freedom in that they are free to think. It is the exploration of this thought and of feeling, that can form the basis of much counselling in this field.

Some nurses and other health professionals may be guilty of overstating the autonomy of the people for whom they care but this is unlikely to be the case with forensic psychiatric nurses who necessarily have a limited amount of freedom.

Directive counselling

Traditionally, and before the client-centred approach was developed, it was more usual to seek advice from counsellors. Directive counselling is the exact opposite to the client-centred approach. It is the process of making suggestions or offering advice to the other person. It is notable that it has tended to be frowned upon in counselling for the past two decades or so. In a study of nurses' attitudes towards counselling, we found that many nurses see their counselling role as a directive one (Burnard and Morrison 1990). Perhaps, sometimes, it is easier to offer people advice and to make suggestions.

Perhaps the ideal is to be able to work appropriately in both the client-centred and directive modes. One framework for using this balanced approach is Six Category Intervention Analysis (Heron 1990). The analysis is not a particular theory of counselling nor even a specific type of counselling. It does, however, identify a whole range of possible counselling interventions. It is to that analysis that we now turn.

Client-centred and directive: six category intervention analysis

The six categories in Heron's analysis are : prescriptive (offering advice), informative (offering information), confronting (challenging), cathartic (enabling the expression of pent-up emotions), catalytic ('drawing out') and supportive (confirming or encouraging) (Heron 1990). The word 'intervention' is used to describe any statement that the counsellor may use. The word 'category' is used to denote a range of related interventions.

Heron calls the first three categories of intervention, (prescriptive, informative and confronting),'authoritative' and suggests that in using these categories the nurse retains control over the relationship. He calls the second three categories of intervention (cathartic, catalytic and supportive), 'facilitative' and suggests that these enable the client to retain control over the relationship. In other words, the first three are 'nurse-centred' and the second three are 'client-centred'. Another way of describing the difference between the first and second sets of three categories is that the first three are 'You tell me' interventions and the second three are 'I tell you' interventions.

What, then, is the value of such an analysis of therapeutic interventions? First. it identifies the range of possible interventions available to the nurse/counsellor. Very often, in day to day interactions with others, we stick to repetitive forms of conversation and response simply because we are not aware that other options are available to us. This analysis identifies an exhaustive range of types of human interventions. Second, by identifying the sorts of interventions we can use, we can act more precisely and with a greater sense of intention. The nurse/patient relationship thus becomes more particular and less haphazard : we know what we are saying and also how we are saying it. We have greater interpersonal choice.

Third, the analysis offers an instrument for training. Once the categories have been identified, they can be used for students and others to identify their weaknesses and strengths across the interpersonal spectrum Nurses can, in this way, develop a wide range and comprehensive range of interpersonal skills. Heron's six category analysis has been adopted widely in nursing colleges as the means of training people to develop their interpersonal skills.

In two research studies, we invited both student nurses and trained nursing staff to identify their own strengths and weaknesses in terms of the Six Category Intervention Analysis (Burnard and Morrison 1988, Morrison and Burnard 1989). In the first study, using an convenience sample of 92 trained nurses, those nurses were asked to rank order the six categories according how skilful they thought they were in using them. Generally speaking the nurses perceived themselves to be more skilled in using the authoritative categories and less skilled in using the facilitative categories. Having said that, most of the nurses perceived themselves as being particularly weak in using cathartic and catalytic interventions. Overall, they perceived themselves as being best at being supportive.

There were marked similarities in the findings of the second study in which we invited 84 student nurses to rank order the six categories in terms of their perceived strengths and weaknesses in using them. Again we found an overall picture of greater perceived skill in using authoritative interventions rather than facilitative ones. Students also thought that they were generally most effective in using supportive interventions and not so good at using cathartic and confronting interventions. In general, the results of both studies support Heron's (1990) assertion that a wide range of nurses in our society show a much greater deficit in the skilful use of facilitative interventions that they do in the skilful use of authoritative ones.

These findings suggest that there is still much to be done to help nurses to be more client-centred. They appear to be quite good at being authoritative and advice-giving. If they are to be good all-rounders in the field of counselling, it seems to be important to develop the catalytic, confronting and cathartic elements of Heron's analysis.

Which should forensic nurses use?

In the last two decades, the accent, in counselling, has tended to be on the client-centred sort. The prevailing wisdom has it that most counsellors should listen to their clients, encourage them to identify their own problems and seek their own solutions. On the other hand, as we have seen, there are occasions in nursing and in medicine, where advice and prescription are necessary. The nurse is likely to be most skilled if she is able to move freely and appropriately between both types of counselling. Unfortunately, though, this can sometimes mean that the slide is towards the more authoritative and nurse-centred sort of counselling. It would appear that, given the choice, nurses tend towards being prescriptive rather than facilitative.

No doubt there are many reasons for this. Nurse training, until fairly recently, has tended to be prescriptive so it is hardly surprising that nurse, themselves, become prescriptive. Also, nursing is a highly practical profession which aims at problem resolution. It may, at times, seem easier to offer advice as a means of finding quick solutions to difficult problems. Finally, in this short list of possibilities, many nurses are taught to observe patients for signs and symptoms and then to act on what they observe. This is quite different to the client-centred approach to counselling. In that sort of counselling, the nurse is required to get to know the patient as the patient sees him or herself. The nurse is not required merely to observe, report and act. She must get to know the patient from the patient's point of view. This means a considerable change of direction. However, if nursing practice is to develop and grow, it is a change that is worth making. It is clear, too, that the forensic nurse is likely to need to offer a balanced approach to counselling: the client-centred approach balanced by and with the more directive approach.

These ideas, then, may serve as a catalyst for thinking about the extended or expanded role of the forensic nurse. It is likely, of course, that many forensic nurses already function as counsellors and develop therapeutic relationships with their client. It seems likely, too, that a number do not. Perhaps future training courses for forensic psychiatric nurses could include the development of counselling skills as part of a range of therapeutic skills that are available to all those who work in controlled environments. Many more books and papers that refer to these sorts of developments are included in the bibliography of this book. It would seem that if forensic psychiatric nursing is to grow and prosper, the therapeutic role of the nurse is the way in which the role may be expanded.

Conclusion

This book has offered something of a beginning. The studies reported here are all small scale ones and their findings cannot be generalised to a larger populations. We have resisted drawing any conclusions about the national picture, based on the findings reported here. On the other hand, the studies do offer insights into the ways in which some forensic psychiatric nurses view aspects of their jobs. They also represent a beginning: a tentative move towards researching an under-researched field. Lots more has to be done. First, and perhaps taking a lead from some of the studies here, there needs to be a well thought out and properly financed research programme that will seek to find out what it is that forensic psychiatric nurses do. This would seem to be the first step: to define the field. Then, further studies might explore what it is that forensic nurses do that is *therapeutic*. In the larger psychiatric nursing arena, much emphasis has been placed on the idea that what those nurses do should be of therapeutic value (although there is still little empirical work to indicate whether or not this really is the case). Although forensic work is a speciality, it would seem reasonable to suggest that the work of nurses in this field should also have a therapuetic value. Finally, in the short list of what might be done in the future, it would seem important that some *consumer* studies be carried out. What do the people who receive the ministrations of forensic psychiatric nurses feel about the care (or otherwise) that they receive? Again, in both general and psychiatric nursing, there have been few such studies.

All of this sort of research should lead us to greater clarity in two aspects of the field. First, it should help in making decisions about how best to provide for and care for the forensic patient or client. Second, it should offer guidance about how best to train forensic psychiatric nurses. Whilst a range of trainining initiatives exist for forensic nurses, none of these appears to have arisen out of rigourous research projects. We hope, then, that the studies described and discussed in this book will offer ideas for the next stage in the enterprise: the more detailed mapping out and describing of what is, at once, an interesting and a neglected field of study.

References

Aldridge, D. (1988) Treating self-mutilatory behaviour: A Social Strategy, *Family Systems Medicine* 6:1, 5 - 20.

Ashton, J. (1986) Preventing Suicide in Hospital *Nursing Times*, 82, 52, 36-37.

Aston, A. & Thomas, L. (1987) Mother And Baby Facilities In England and Wales 1985-1986. *Marce Society Bulletin*, 3-12.

Bach-Y-Rita, G. (1974) Habitual violence and self-mutilation, *American Journal of Psychiatry*. 131:9, 1018 - 1020.

Bardon, D.A. (1977) Mother And Baby Unit In A Psychiatric Hospital. *Nursing Mirror* 145, 30-33.

Bardon D, Glaser, Y.I.M. Prothero, D. & Weston D.H. (1968) The Mother And Baby Unit: A Psychiatric Survey Of 115 Cases. *British Medical Journal*. 2:775-758.

Barraclough, J.B. (1974) A Hundred Cases of Suicide : Clinical Aspects *British Journal of Psychiatry*, 124, 355-373.

Blade, P. (1977) The Clinical Specialist as Nurse Consultant Journal of *Nursing Administration*, 7: 33-36.

Blythe, M.M. and Pearlmutter, D.R (1983) The Suicide Watch: A Re-Examination of Maximum Observation, *Perspectives In Psychiatric Care*, 11, 3, 90-93.

Brandit, R.B. (1975) *The Morality and Rationality of Suicide*: Oxford University Press, Oxford.

Broadmoor Hospital (1989) *Observation of Patients* Clinical Nursing Policies and Procedures, Broadmoor Hospital.

Browne, A. Finkelhor, D. (1986) Impact of child sexual abuse: A review of the research, *Psychological Bulletin* 99:1.

Bunsteed, E.L. and Johnstone, C. (1983) The Development of Suicide Precautions for an In-Patient Psychiatric Unit, *Journal of Psychological Nursing and Mental Health Services*, 21, 5, 15-109.

Burnard, P. and Morrison, P. (1989) Client-Centred Approach: *Nursing Times* : 85 : 15 : 60 - 61.

Burnard, P. (1990) *Experential Learning in Action*: Avebury, Aldershot.

Burnard, P. and Morrison, P. (1992) *Self-Disclosure: a Contemporary Analysis*: Avebury, Aldershot.

Burnard, P. and Morrison, P. (1987) Nurses' Perceptions of Their Own Interpersonal Skills, *Nursing Times*, 83 : 42 : 59.

Burrow, S. (1992) The deliberate self-harming behaviour of patients within a British special hospital, *Journal of Advanced Nursing 17*, 138 - 148.

Butler Committee (1975) *Report On The Committee of Mentally Disordered Offenders*, HMSO London.

Carmen, E., Reiker, P., Mills, T. (1984) Victims of violence and psychiatric illness, *American Journal of Psychiatry*, 141:3 378 - 383.

Chandler, S.E. (1990) *Hospital Fire Statistics - An analysis of recent trends*, Building Research Establishment. PD 111/89. Borehamwood Wood.

Clarke A.L. (1976) Recognising Discord Between Mother And Child And Changing it to Harmony. *American Journal of Maternal Child Nursing*, 12, 100-106

Cookson, H.M. (1977) A survey of self-injury in a closed prison for women, *British Journal of Criminology* 17:4 332 - 346.

Copas, J.B. and Robin A. (1982) Suicide in psychiatric In-patients. *British Journal of Psychiatry*, 141, 503-511.

Cox, M. (1990) *Structuring the Therapeutic Process*, Jessica Kingsley, London.

Crabtree, M. S. (1979) Effective Utilization of Clinical Specialists within the Organisation Structure of Hospital Nursing Service, *Nursing Administration Quarterly* 4,1, 1-11.

Crammer, J.L. (1984) The Special Characteristics of Suicide in Hospital In-Patients, *British Journal of Psychiatry*, 145, 460-476.

Daldin, H. (1988) A contribution to the understanding of self-mutilating behaviour in adolescence. *Journal of Child Psychotherapy*, 14, 16-66.

Department of Health and Social Security (1983) *The Mental Health Act.* DHSS, London.

Department of Health and Social Security (1983) *Draft code of practice.* The Mental Health Act. DHSS, London.

Department of Health and Social Security (1959) *The Mental Health Act.* DHSS, London.

DeWitt. K. (1900) Speciality in Nursing, *American Journal of Nursing*, 1, 14-17.

Diggory, J. C. (1974) *Basic Research Issues in Suicide*, Charles Press, New York.

Diggory, J. C. (1974) *Will 'O the Wisp of Reasonable Challenge*, Charles Press, New York.

Dooley, E. (1990) Prison Suicide in England and Wales 1972 *British Journal of Psychiatry*, 156, 40-45.

Dooley, E. (1990) Unnatural Deaths in Prison, *British Journal of Criminology*, 30, 2, 229-234.

Dooley, E. (1990) Prison Suicide in England and Wales, *British Journal of Psychiatry*: 156, 40-45.

Dorpat, T. and Ripely, H.S. (1977) A study of suicides in the Seattle Area. *Comprehensive Psychiatry*, 1, 349-59.

Douglas G. (1956) Psychotic Mothers. *Lancet* Jan 21, 124-125.

DSM III (1980) *Diagnostic and Statistical Manual of Mental Disorders*. Third Edition, American Psychiatric Association. Washington D.C.

Eisenberg, M.G. (1990) Detection of Suicide Risk Among Hospitalised Veterans *Journal of Rehabilitation*, 56, 1, 63-68.

Everson, S. (1981) The Integration of the Role of the CNS Journal of *Continuing Education Nursing*, 12, 2, 16-19.

Farberow, N.L. (1967) *Essays in self destruction*, Aronson, New York: Aronson.

Faulk, M.(1988) *Basic Forensic Psychiatry*, Blackwell Scientific, London.

Favazza, A. Conterio, K. (1988) The plight of chronic self-mutilators, *Community Mental Health Journal* 24:1 22 - 30.

Fenton, M. (1985) Identity Competencies of the CNS, *Journal of Nursing Administration*, 13, 4, 14-17.

Fernando, S, and Storm, V. (1984) Suicide among psychiatric patients of a District General Hospital, *Psychological Medicine.* 14, 661-672.

Forgas, J. P. (1985) *Interpersonal Behaviour: The psychology of social interaction.* Pergamon, London.

Franklin, R. (1988) Deliberate self-harm - self injurious behaviour within a correctional mental health, *Criminal Justice and Behaviour* 15:2 210 - 218.

Frickman L.E.(1973) Hospital Fires: Preparing Staff before one starts, *Hospital and Community Psychiatry* 24, 1, 23-32.

Gale, S. (1980) A Study of Suicide in State Mental Hospitals in New York City, *Psychiatric Quarterly* 52, 201-213

Gardner, A.R. and Gardner, A.J. (1975) Self mutilation, obsessionality and narcissism, *British Journal of Psychiatry* 127, 127 - 132.

Gaston, E.H. (1982) Solving the Smoking Problem on a Chronic Ward, *Journal of Psychiatric Treatment and Evaluation*, 4, 5, 397-401.

Geller, J.L. & Bertsch, G. (1985) Fire Setting Behaviour in the Histories of a State Hospital Population, *American Journal of Psychiatry* 142, 4, 464-468.

Gibson, B. (1989) The use of seclusion, *Nursing*, 3, 43.

Glancy Report (1973) *Report on Security in NHS Hospitals*, DHSS, London.

Goffman, I. (1961) *Asylums*, Pelican, Harmondsworth.

Goldberg, R.J. (1989) The use of Constant Observation in General Hospitals, *International Journal of Psychiatry in Medicine*, 19, 2, 193-201.

Gordon, M. (1969) The Clinical Specialist as Change Agent, *Nursing Outlook*, 17, 3, 37-39.

Gostin, L. (1985) *Secure provision. A review of special services for the mentally ill and mentally handicapped in England and Wales.* Tavistock, London.

Graff, M. and Mallin, R. (1967) The syndrome of the wrist cutter, *American Journal of Psychiatry* 124:1, 36 - 42.

Green, A. (1978) Self-destructive behaviour in battered children, *American Psychiatric Association* 135:5.

Griffin, W. (1989) An Act of Suicide : Did You Hear The Cry? *Canadian Journal of Psychiatric Nursing*, 30, 3, 14-16.

Grounds, A. (1990) Seclusion. In: Bluglass, R.,Bowden, P. *Principles and Practice of Forensic Psychiatry.* Edinburgh, Churchill Livingstone. ✓

Guze, P. and Robins, R. (1970) Suicide and Primary Affective Disorders. *British Journal Psychiatry*, 117, 437-8.

Hagnell, O. and Rorsam, B. (1978) Suicide and endogenous depression with some somatic systems in the Lundby study, *Neuropsychobiolical Journal*, 4, 180-187.

Hamil, K. (1987) Seclusion: Inside looking out, *Nursing Times*, 4, 38-39.

Hamric A (1983) *Role, Development and Functions in the Clinical Nurse Specialist in Theory and in Practice*, Grune and Stratton, New York.

Hardek, E.A. (1988) Crisis Intervention and Suicide *Journal of*

Psychological Nursing, 26, 5, 24-27.

Harris, G.T. & Rice, M.E. (1984) Mentally Disordered Fire Setters: Psychodynamic versus Empirical Approaches, *International Journal of Law and Psychiatry,* 7, 19-34 .

Hawkins, P. and Shohet, R. (1989) *Supervision and the Helping Professions,* Open University Press, Milton Keynes

Hawton, K. (1987) Assessment of Suicide Risk, *British Journal of Psychiatry,* 151, 145-153.

Heron, J. (1990) *Helping the Client,* Sage, London.

Hill, R.W., Langevin, R., Paitich, D., Handy L., Russon, A. & Wilkinson, L. (1982) Is Arson an Aggressive Act or a Property Offence? A Controlled Study of Psychiatric Referrals, *Canadian Journal of Psychiatry* 27, 648-654.

Hodgeman, E. (1983) The CNS as Researcher, *Journal of Nursing Education,* 25, 4-9.

Hodgkinson, P.E. (1985) The use of seclusion. *Medicine, Science and the Law,* 25, 3, 215-222.

Holley, H. & Arboleda-Florez, J.E. (1988) Hypernomia and Self-Destructiveness in Penal Settings, *International Journal of Law and Psychiatry,* 11, 168-178.

Howard League (1990) *Briefing Paper: Women And Children In Prison,* Howard League, London.

Hunter, T. and Russel, C. (1990) *Managing Health Services.* Book 4. Choosing and developing your team, Open University, Milton Keynes.

Hurley, W. & Monahan, T.M. (1969) Arson; The Criminal and The Crime, *British Journal of Criminology,* 9, 4-21.

Jackson, B. (1973) Hospital Administrators must know about Clinical Specialists, *Supervisor Nurse*, 5, 29-35.

Jackson, H.F., Glass, C. & Hope, S. (1987) A Functional Analysis of Recidivist Arson, *British Journal of Clinical Psychology*, 26, 175-185.

Jackson H.F., Hope S. & Glass C. (1987) Why are Arsonists not Violent Offenders? *International Journal of Offender Therapy and Comparative Criminology* 31, 3, 143-151.

Jacobs, F.G. (1975) *The European Convention on Human Rights*, Clarendon Press, Oxford.

Jacobson, R., Jackson, M. & Berelowitz, M. (1986) Self Incineration: A Controlled Comparison of In-patient Suicide Attempts. Clinical Features and History of Self Harm, *Psychological Medicine*, 16, 107-116.

Kafka, J. (1969) The body as a transitional object: A psychoanalytic study of a self mutilating patient, *British Journal of Medical Psychology* 42, 207 - 212.

Kafry, D. (1980) Playing with Matches: Children and Fires, In Canter, D. (ed) *Fires and Human Behaviour*, Wiley, Chichester.

Kelly, G. (1963) *A Theory of Personality*, Norton, New York.

Kerrane, T. (1975) The Clinical Nurse Specialist, *Nursing Mirror*, 30 63-65.

Kessel, N. and McCulloch, W. (1966) Repeated acts of self poisoning and self injury, *Proceedings of the Royal Society of Medicine*, 59, 89-92.

Kibbee, P. (1988) The Suicidal Patient An Issue for Quality Assurance and Risk Management, *Journal of Nursing Quality Assurance*, 3, 1, 63-71.

Kitchiner, N. et al (1992)   The role of the forensic psychiatric nurse, *Nursing Times*. 88, 8.

Koson, D.F. & Dvoskin, H.   (1982)   Arson; A Diagnostic Study, *Bulletin of the American Academy of Psychiatry and Law*, 10, 1, 39-49.

Kumar, R., Meltzer, E.S., Hepplewhite, R. & Stephenson, A.D. (1986) Admitting Mentally Ill Mothers With Their Babies into Psychiatric Hospitals, *Bulletin of the Royal College of Psychiatrists*, 10, 169-172.

Langley, G.E. Bayatti, N.N. (1984) Suicide In Exe Vale Hospital *British Journal of Psychiatry*, 145, 460-476.

Leopoldt, H. (1985) A secure and secluded spot, *Nursing Times*, 6, 26-28.

Lester, D. (1972) Self mutilating behaviour, *Psychological Bulletin* 78:2 119 - 128.

Leupher, E.T. (1972) Joint Admission And Evaluation Of Post-Partum Psychiatric Patients And Their Infants, *Hospital And Community Psychiatry*, 23, 284-286.

Levey, S. (1990) *Suicide: Principles and Practice of Forensic Psychiatry,* Churchill Livingstone, Edinburgh.

Lyttle, J. (1986) *Mental Disorder*, Balliere Tindall, London.

MacDonald, A. (1988) Changing professional practice, *Senior Nurse*, 8, 11, 4-7.

Main, F.T. & Durh, M.D.   (1958)   Mothers With Children In A Psychiatric Hospital, *Lancet*, 18 124-125.

Mallison, M. (1984) The Shoes of the Clinician, *The American Journal of Nursing* 84, 587.

Mansell, K. (1984) Mother Baby Unit: The concept works, *Maternal Child Nursing*, 9, 132-133.

Marjolis, P.M. (1965) *Suicide Precautions*, Permagon Press, Oxford.

Mason, W. and Sponholz, R. (1963) Behaviour or rhesus monkeys weaned in isolation, *Journal of Psychiatric Research*, 1, 299-306.

McCoy, S.M. and Garritson, S. (1983) Seclusion, the process of intervening, *Journal of Psychosocial Nursing and Mental Health Services*, 21, 8, 8-15.

McCulloch, J. and Phillip, A. (1972) *Suicidal Behaviour*, Pergamon Press, Oxford.

McKerracher, D., Loughnane, T. and Watson, R. (1968) Self mutilating in female psychopaths, *British Journal of Psychiatry*, 114, 829 - 832.

Mead, M. (1950) *Male and Female*, Pelican, Harmondsworth.

Metcalf, J. Werner, M. and Richmond, T. (1984) The CNS in a Clinical Career Ladder, *Nursing Administration Quarterly*, 9,3, 9-19.

Modestin, J. (1986) *Why People Kill Themselves*, Second Edition, Thomas Springfield, Illinois.

Modestine, J. and Wurmle, O. (1989) Role of Modelling in In-Patient Suicide : A Lack of Supporting Evidence, *British Journal of Psychiatry*, 154, 511-514.

Morgan, H.G. (1979) *Death Wishes? The Understanding and Management of Deliberate Self Harm*, Wiley, Chichester.

Morgan, H.G. and Priest, P. (1984) Assessment of Suicide Risk in Psychiatric In-patients, *British Journal of Psychiatry*, 145, 460-476.

Morrison, P. (1987) The practice of seclusion. *Nursing Times*, 83:19, 62-66.

Morrison, P. and Burnard, P. (1990) *Caring and Communicating: The Therapeutic Relationship in Nursing*: Macmillan, Basingstoke.

Mortality Statistics (1985) - HMSO, London.

Motto Jerome, A.M.D. (1974) *Refinement of Variables in Assessing Suicide: Issues Concerning Research in Suicide Prevention*, Charles Press, New York.

Murgatroyd, S. (1985) *Counselling and Helping*, Methuen, London.

Niskala, H. (1984) Competencies and Skills required by Nurses working in Forensic Areas, *Western Journal of Nursing Research*, 8, 4, 400-413.

Niskala, H. (1986) Competencies and skills required by nurses working in forensic areas, *Western Journal of Nursing Research*, 8, 4, 400-413.

Niskanen, P. (1975) Suicide in Helsinki Psychiatric Hospitals, *Psychiatria Fennica*, 275-280.

O'Gorman, G. (1976) Means of restraint, *Nursing Times*, 72, 20, 785.

O'Sullivan, G.H. & Kelleher M. (1987) A Study of Fire Setters in the South-West of Ireland, *British Journal of Psychiatry*, 151, 818-823.

Oakley, A. (1981) Mothers & children in society, *Nursing*, 21, 896-901.

Pallis, D.J. and Birtchnell, J. (1977) Seriousness of suicide attempt in relation to personality, *British Journal of Psychiatry*, 130, 252-259.

Parry, J. (1991) Community Care for Mentally Ill Offenders, *Nursing Standard*, 5, 23, 29-33.

Patterson, C.H. (1985) *The Therapeutic Relationship : Foundations for an eclectic psychotherapy*, Brooks/Cole, Pacific Grove, California.

Pederson, P. (1988) The role of community psychiatric nurses in forensic psychiatric, *Community Psychiatric Nurses Journal*, June, 12 - 17.

Peplau, H. (1965) Specialisation and Professional Nursing, *Nursing Science*, August, 268-298.

Perry, L. (1991) Burning Anger, *Nursing Times*, 87, 23, 38-40.

Pfeffer, C.R. (1983) 138 Suicidal behaviour in children. A review with implications for research and practice, *American Journal Psychiatry.* 138, 154-159.

Phillips, M. S. (1983) Forensic psychiatry - Nurses attitude revealed, *Dimensions.* 60, 9. 41-43.

Phillips, M. S. (1980) Forensic psychiatric programme for nurses, *Dimensions.* 43, 6, 29-30.

Phillips, R. and Alkan, M. (1961) Some Aspects of self-mutilation in the general population of a large psychiatric hospital, *Psychiatric Quarterly*, 35, 421-423.

Pillette, P.C. (1978) The tyranny of seclusion: A brief essay, *Journal of Psychiatric Nursing*, l6, 10, 19-21.

Pokornay, A.D. (1964) Suicide rates in various psychiatric disorders, *Journal of nervous and mental disease*, 139, 499-506.

Power, K.G. & Spencer, A.P. (1987) Parasuicidal Behaviour of Detained Scottish Young Offenders, *International Journal of Offender Therapy and Comparative Criminology*, 31, 227-235.

Prins, H., Tennent, G. & Trick, K. (1985) Motives for Arson, *Medicine, Science and Law*, 25, 4, 275-278.

Quinn, S. (1979) Management of an interim secure unit, *Nursing Times*, Feb. 9, 237-240.

RCN (1988) *Specialities in Nursing*, RCN, London.

RCN Society of Psychiatric Nursing. (1979) *Seclusion and Restraint in Hospitals and Units for the Mentally Disordered*, Royal College of Nursing, 2.

Resnik, H.L.P. (1974) Psychological resynthesis. A clinical approach to the survivors of a death by suicide, *Hospitals and community psychiatry*, 25, 33-36.

Rice, M.E. & Chaplin, T.C. (1979) Social Skills Training for Hospitalized Male Arsonists, *Journal of Behaviour Therapy and Experimental Psychiatry*, 10 105-108.

Ritter, S. (1989) *Manual of Clinical Psychiatric Nursing Principles and Procedures*, Harper and Row, New London.

Rix, G. & Seymour, D. (1988) Violent Incidents on a regional secure unit, *Journal of Advanced Nursing*, 13 746-751.

Rogers, C.R. (1964) *On Becoming a Person*: Constable, London.

Ropka, M. and Fay, F. (1984) CNS - Alive and Well?, *American Journal of Nursing* 84, 661-664

Rosen, G. (1975) *History of Suicide*, Oxford University Press, Oxford.

Rosenstock, H.A., Holland, M.A. & Jones, P.H. (1980) Fire-setting on an Adolescent Inpatient Unit: An Analysis, *Journal of Clinical Psychiatry* 41, 1, 20-22 .

Rosenthal, T.T. & Rosenthal, S.L. (1988) Foresight - Secret of Survival, *Nursing Management* 19, 5, 80.

Rosenthal, R. et al (1972) Wrist cutting syndrome: The meaning of a gesture, *American Journal of Psychiatry* 128:11 1363 - 68.

Ross, R. and McKay, H. (1979) *Self-mutilation*, Lexington Books, Toronto.

Roy, A. (1978) Self-mutilation *British Journal of Medical Psychology* 51, 201 - 203.

Roy, A. (1982) Suicide in chronic schizophrenia, *British Journal of Psychiatry*, 141, 171-177.

Russell, D., Hodgkinson, P., and Hillis, J.A. (1986) Time Out, *Nursing Times*, Feb 26, 47-49.

Salmons, P.H., and Whittington, R.M. (1989) Hospital suicides: Are there preventable factors?, *British Journal of Psychiatry*, 154, 247-249.

Salmons, P.H. (1984) Suicide in High Buildings, *British Journal of Psychiatry* 145, 460-476.

Sapsford, R.J., Banks, C. & Smith, D.P. (1978) Arsonists in Prison, *Medicine, Science and Law,* 18,4, 247-254.

Schaeffer, C., Carroll, J. and Abramowitz, S. (1982) Self mutilation and the borderline personality, *The Journal of Neurons and Mental Disease* 170:8, 468 - 473.

Service Establishments in England and Wales, HMSO, London.

Shapiro, S. (1987) Self-mutilation and self-blame in incest victims, *American Journal of Psychotherapy* XLI:I, 46 - 54.

Shapiro, S. and Waltzer, H. (1980) Successful suicides and serious attempts in a General Hospital over a fifteen year period, *General Hospital Psychiatry,* 2, 118-126.

Shneidman, E.S. (1981) The psychological autopsy, *Suicide and Life Threatening Behaviour,* 11, 325-340.

Simpson, C. (1981) Self-mutilation in children and adolescents, *Bulletin of the Menninger Clinic* 45:5, 428 - 438.

Slater, P. (1977) *Dimension of Inter-personal Space*, Wiley, London.

Sletten, I. (1972) Suicides in Mental hospital patients, *Diseases of the Nervous System*, 29, 328-334.

Sneddon, J. Kerry. R, & Bant. W. (1981) The Psychiatric Mother and baby unit. A Three Year Study, *The Practitioner*, 225, 1295-1300.

Soloff, P.H. and Turner, S.M. (1981) Patterns of seclusion: A prospective study, *Journal of Nervous Mental Disorders*, 169, l, 37.

Soni-Raliegh, V., Bulusu, L. & Balarajan, R. (1990) Suicide Among Immigrants from the Indian Sub-Continent, *British Journal of Psychiatry*, 156, 46-50

Soothill, K. (1990) Arson. In Bluglass, R. & Bowden, P. *Principles and Practise of Forensic Psychiatry*, Churchill Livingstone, Edinburgh.

Stafford. R, (1991) The Evolution of the Specialist, *Nursing Times*, April 17-23, 39-40.

Stengle, E. (1964) *Suicide and Attempted Suicide*, Penguin, Harmondsworth.

Stollard, P. (1984) A system for the Analysis of Fire reports, and It's Application to Health Care Buildings, *Fire Safety Journal*, 8, 169-175.

Stollard, P. (1983) The Codification and Interpretation of Hospital Fire Reports, *Health Bulletin*, 41, 5, 238-247.

Stollard, P. (1984) An Analysis of Hospital Fire reports. *Health Trends* 16, 71-72.

Tangari, A. (1974) Family Involvement In The Treatment of a Psychiatric Inpatient, *Hospital And Community Psychiatry*, 25, 792-794.

Tarbuck, P. (1990) *Curriculum for the E.N.B. 770, Nursing in controlled environments course*, Ashworth Hospital.

Tardiff, K. (1980) Assault, Suicide and Mental Illness, *Archives of General Psychiatry*, 37, 164-169.

Tardiff, K. (1981) Emergency control measures for psychiatric in-patients, *Journal of Nervous Mental Disorders*, 169, 1, 614.

Taristano, B. (1986) A Demystification of the Clinical Nurse Specialist Role, *The Journal of Nursing Education* 25, 4-9.

Tenroach, K. (1964) Suicide rates among current and former mental institution patients, *Journal of Nervous and Mental Diseases*, 138, 124-130.

Topp, D.O. (1979) Suicide in Prison Examination of Rates of Suicide in Prison including Factors indicating Cause, *British Journal of Psychiatry*, 134, 24-27.

Tousley, M.M. (1985) Fire on the Unit. *Journal of Psychosocial Nursing and Mental Health Services*, 23, 8, 6-9.

Trimnel, J., Poe, D.S., Adams, C., Jones, N.S & Adams, P. (1989) Admitting Mothers And Their Babies, Dealing With Postpartum Illness On The Ward, *Journal of Psychosocial Nursing*, 27, 6-11.

Tuck, M. (1990) *Home Office Research Study 115 Suicide and Self in Prison*, HMSO, London.

Tumin, S. (1990) *Review of Suicide and Self Harm in Prison*, Tavistock, London.

Vreeland R.G. & Levin B.M. (1980) *Psychological Aspects of Firesetting*. In Canter, D. (ed) *Fires and Human Behaviour*, Wiley, Chichester.

Walde, P.H.V.D., Meeks, D., Gruebaum, H.U., & Weiss J.L. (1968) Joint Admission Of Mothers and Children to a State Hospital, *Archives of General Psychiatry*, 18, 706-711.

Warlingham Park Hospital (1981) *Report into Warlingham Park Hospital Fire*, Croydon Area Health Authority.

Warwick, G. (1983) Mother Baby Separation- One Of The Dangers Of Temporary Separation Caused By The Hospital Admission, *Nursing Times*, 23, 64-67.

Welsh Office (1989) *Mental Illness Services: A Strategy for Wales*, Welsh Office.

White, S. (1987) Mothers In Custody And The Punishment Of Children, *Probation Journal*, 36, 106-109.

Wyatt, D.M. (1985) Are You Prepared for a Hospital Fire?, *Nursing*, 15, 2, 51.

Yesavage, J.A., Benezech, M., Ceccaldi, P., Bourgeois, M. & Addad M. (1983) Arson in Mentally Ill and Criminal Populations, *Journal of Clinical Psychiatry*, 44, 128-130.

Zubin, J. (1974) *Historical and Philosophical Perspectives on Classification of Suicide*, Charles Press, New York.

Bibliography

Argyle, M. (1983) *The Psychology of Interpersonal Behaviour*, 4th Edition, Penguin, Harmondsworth.

Argyle, M (ed) (1981) *Social Skills and Health*, Methuen, London

Arnold, E. and Boggs, K. (1989) *Interpersonal Relationships, Professional Communication Skills for Nurses*, Saunders, Philadelphia

Baruth, L.G. (1987) *An Introduction to the Counselling Profession*, Prentice Hall, Englewood Cliffs, New Jersey

Belkin, G.S.(1984) *Introduction to Counselling*, Brown, Dubuque,Iowa

Bellack, A.S. and Hersen, M. (eds) (1979) *Research and Practice in Social Skills Training*, Plenum Press, New York.

Benner, P. and Wrubel, J. (1989) *The Primacy of Caring, Stress and Coping in Health and Illness*, Addison Wesley, Menlo Park.

Bolger, A.W. (ed) (1982) *Counselling in Britain, a reader*, Batsford Academic, London.

Boud, D., Keogh, R. and Walker, M. (1985) *Reflection, Turning Experience into Learning*, Kogan Page, London.

Boud, D.J. (ed) (1981) *Developing Student Autonomy in Learning*, Kogan Page, London.

Bower, S.A. and Bower, G.H. (1976), *Asserting Yourself*, Addison Wesley, Reading, Mass.

Broome, A. (1990) *Managing Change*, Macmillan, London.

Brown, D. and Srebalus, D. J. (1988) *An Introduction to the Counselling Process*, Prentice Hall, Philadelphia, PA.

Calnan, J. (1983) *Talking With Patients*, Heinemann, London.

Campbell, A. (1984) *Paid to Care?* SPCK, London.

Carkuff, R.R. (1969) *Helping and Human Relations, Vol I, Selection and Training*, Holt, Rinehart and Winston, New York.

Carlisle, J. and Leary, M. (1982) Negotiating Groups. In Payne, R. and Cooper, C. (eds) *Groups at Work*, Wiley, Chichester.

Chenevert, M. (1978) *Special Techniques in Assertiveness Training for Women in the Health Professions*, C.V. Mosby, St Louis.

Curran, J. and Monti, P. (eds), *Social Skills Training, A Practical Handbook for Assessment and Treatment*, Guildford, New York.

Dryden, W., Charles-Edwards, D. and Woolfe, R. (1989) *Handbook of Counselling in Britain*, Routledge, London.

Duncan, S. and Fiske, D.W. (1977) *Face-to-Face Interaction, Research, Methods and Theory*: Lawrence Erlbaum Associates, Hillsdale, New Jersey.

Evans, D. (ed) (1990) *Why Should We Care?*, Macmillan, London.

Fernando, S. (1990) *Mental Health, Race and Culture*, Macmillan, London.

Filley, A.C. (1975) *Interpersonal Conflict Resolution*, Scott, Foresman, Glenview, Illinois.

Fineman, S. (1985) *Social Work Stress and Intervention*, Gower, London.

Firth, H., McKeown, P., McIntee, J. and Britton, P. (1987) Burn-Out, Personality and Support in Long-Stay Nursing, *Nursing Times*, 83, 32, 55 - 57.

Glennerster, H. and Owens, P. (1990) *Nursing in Conflict*, Macmillan, London.

Goffman, I. (1971) *The Presentation of Self in Everyday Life*, Penguin, Harmondsworth.

Graham, N.M. (1988) Psychological Stress as a Public Health Problem: How Much Do We Know?, *Community Health Studies*, 12, 2, 151-160.

Haggerty, L.A. (1987) An Analysis of Senior Nursing Students' Immediate Responses to Distressed Patients, *Journal of Advanced Nursing*, 12, 4, 451 - 461.

Hargie, O. (ed) (1987) *A Handbook of Communication Skills*, Croom Helm, London.

Hargie, O., Saunders, C. and Dickson, D. (1981) *Social Skills in Interpersonal Communication*, 2nd Edition,Croom Helm, London.

Heginbotham, C. (1990) *Mental Health, Human Rights and Legislation*, Macmillan, London.

Hill, S.S. and Howlett, H.A. (1988) *Success in Practical Nursing in Personal Vocational Issues*, W.B. Saunders, Philadelphia, PA.

Hull, D. and Schroeder, H. (1979) Some Interpersonal Effects of Assertion, Non-Assertion and Aggression, *Behaviour Therapy*, 10: 20 -29.

Ivey, A.E.(1987) *Counselling and Psychotherapy, Skills, theories and practice*, Prentice Hall International, London

Jones, J.G., Janman, K., Payne, R.L. and Rick, J.T. (1987) Some Determinants of Stress in Psychiatric Nurses, *International Journal of Nursing Studies*, 24, 2, 129 - 144.

Kilty, J. (1987) *Staff Development for Nurse Education, Practitioners Supporting Students, A Report of a 5-Day Development Workshop*, Human Potential Research Project, University of Surrey, Guildford.

Larson, D.G. (1986) Developing Effective Hospice Staff Support Groups, Pilot Test of an Innovative Training Programs, *Hospice Journal*, 2, 2, 41 - 55.

Lyon, B.L. and Werner, J.S. (1987) Research on Nursing Practice, Stress, *Annual Review of Nursing Research*, 5, 3-22.

Morrison, P. and Burnard, P. (1988) Clarifying Nurses' Interpersonal Skills, *Nursing Times*, 84, 30, 49.

Morrison, P. and Burnard, P. (1989) Students' and Trained Nurses' Perceptions of Their Own Interpersonal Skills, a report and comparison, *Journal of Advanced Nursing*, 14, 321 - 329.

Munro, A., Manthei, B. and Small, J.(1988) *Counselling, The Skills of Problem-Solving*, Routledge, London.

Murgatroyd, S. and Woolfe, R. (1982) *Coping with Crisis-Understanding and Helping Persons in Need*, Harper and Row, London.

Myerscough, P.R.(1989) *Talking With Patients, A Basic Clinical Skill* Oxford Medical Publications, Oxford.

Nadler, L. (ed) (1984) *The Handbook of Human Resource Development*, Wiley, New York.

Nelson-Jones, R. (1984) *Personal Responsibility: counselling and therapy, an integrative approach*, Harper and Row, London.

Nelson-Jones, R. (1988) *Practical Counselling and Helping Skills: helping clients to help themselves*, Cassell, London

Nelson, M.J. (1989) *Managing Health Professionals*, Chapman and Hall, London.

Open University Coping With Crisis Group (1987) *Running Workshops, A Guide for Trainers in the Helping Professions*, Croom Helm, London.

Porritt, L. (1990) *Interaction Strategies, An Introduction for Health Professionals*, 2nd Edition, Churchill Livingstone, Edinburgh.

Scammell, B. (1990) *Communication Skills*, Macmillan, London.

Schafer, B.P. and Morgan, M.K. (1980) An Experiential Learning Laboratory, A New Dimension in Teaching Mental Health Skills, *Issues in Mental Health Nursing*, 2, 3, 47 - 57.

Schon, D.A.(1983) *The Reflective Practitioner, How Professionals Think in Action*, Basic Books, New York.

Schulman, D. (1982) *Intervention in Human Services, A guide to skills and knowledge*, 3rd Edition, C.V. Mosby, St Louis, Missouri.

Trower, P. (ed) (1984) *Radical Approaches to Social Skills Training*, Croom Helm, London.

Trower, P., O'Mahony, J.M. and Dryden, W. (1982) Cognitive aspects of social failure, Some implications for social skills training, *British Journal of Guidance and Counselling*, 10, 176 - 184.

Index

181

UU460 MOR X